Three-Dimensional Analysis of Rare Facial Clefts and Clinical Facial Appearance

Three-Dimensional Analysis of Rare Facial Clefts and Clinical Facial Appearance

By

Priscila Padilha Moura,
Roseli Maria Zechi-Ceide,
Antonio Richieri-Costa,
Adriano Porto Peixoto,
Cristiano Tonello
and Daniela Garib

Cambridge Scholars Publishing

Three-Dimensional Analysis of Rare Facial Clefts and Clinical Facial Appearance

By Priscila Padilha Moura, Roseli Maria Zechi-Ceide, Antonio Richieri-Costa, Adriano Porto Peixoto, Cristiano Tonello and Daniela Garib

This book first published 2023

Cambridge Scholars Publishing

Lady Stephenson Library, Newcastle upon Tyne, NE6 2PA, UK

British Library Cataloguing in Publication Data
A catalogue record for this book is available from the British Library

ISBN (10): 1-5275-5226-8
ISBN (13): 978-1-5275-5226-5

For everyone born with some type of orofacial cleft.

TABLE OF CONTENTS

PREFACE

The Hospital for Rehabilitation of Craniofacial Anomalies, University of São Paulo (HRCA/USP) is recognized by the World Health Organization as a "world reference" in craniofacial anomalies care (Freitas et al. 2012). Over 55 years have been dedicated to the multidisciplinary care of individuals with orofacial clefts, including cleft lip and palate, cleft palate, rare facial clefts, craniosynostosis, craniofacial midline anomalies with ocular hypotelorism and hypertelorism, anomalies of the first and second branchial arches, hearing impairment and other complex craniofacial anomalies. Rare facial clefts, also called Tessier clefts, may be isolated or associated with other craniofacial, skeletal or systemic abnormalities. It is not uncommon to observe a combination of multiple rare facial clefts in the same individual, classified as complex cases of rare facial clefts. Most of these cases require a long and costly rehabilitation process, which impacts the affected individual's social, neuropsychological and academic development. This book aims to contribute to the different specialities involved in rare facial cleft care by presenting a three-dimensional representation of craniofacial clefts of 0 to 14 and 30 in the Tessier classification using the presentation of clinical cases of individuals followed up at HRCA/USP. The description of anatomical variations illustrated by photographic images and three-dimensional images from computed tomography reconstruction allows the reader to understand better the craniofacial structures involved in each type of cleft and their phenotypic variations and associations with other rare facial clefts. Visualizing a relationship between tissue changes and bone changes is also possible. We, the authors, hope that a better knowledge of the morphology of rare facial clefts will allow the establishment of personalized and individualized therapeutic practices in high-complexity cases. Thus, recognising repetitive patterns can assist in a more accurate syndromic diagnosis. It will also assist the rehabilitation team in predicting the risks and benefits of therapeutic procedures.

—Freitas, José Alberto de Souza, Lucimara Teixeira das Neves, Ana Lúcia Pompéia Fraga de Almeida, Daniela Gamba Garib, Ivy Kiemle Trindade-Suedam, Renato Yassutaka Faria Yaedú, Rita de Cássia Moura Carvalho Lauris, Simone Soares, Thais Marchini Oliveira and João Henrique Nogueira Pinto. 2012. "Rehabilitative Treatment of Cleft Lip and Palate: Experience of the Hospital for Rehabilitation of

Craniofacial Anomalies/USP (HRAC/USP) - Part 1: Overall Aspects." *Journal of Applied Oral Science* 20 (1): 9–15.

Acknowledgements

This book was developed as a postdoctoral project with the collaboration of an interdisciplinary team under the supervision of a faculty member of our hospital, Dr Daniela Garib (DDS, MSc, PhD, orthodontist). The team included Dr Antonio Richieri-Costa (doctor, geneticist), Dr Roseli Maria Zechi-Ceide (biologist, geneticist), Dr Cristiano Tonello (doctor, craniofacial surgeon), and Dr Adriano Porto Peixoto (DDS, orthodontist). This work has received important support from the researchers of the Department of Clinical Genetics and Molecular Biology of the HRCA-USP (DCGMB-HRCA-USP), mainly Dr Maria Leine Guion-Almeida, Dr Nancy Mizue Kokitsu-Nakata and Dr Siulan Vendramini Paulovich Pittoli, who, together with Dr Antonio Richieri-Costa and Dr Roseli Maria Zechi-Ceide, have been studying patients with rare facial clefts and registering their phenotypes and genetic diagnosis during the thirty years of DCGMB-HRCA-USP's existence. These researchers previously published many of the individual cases presented here, and the references were cited. We thank everyone for their collaboration and contribution to this work.

Affectionately, we thank all the patients and their family members who contributed to the preparation of this work by allowing the use of their images and examinations.

We would like to express our special and sincere thanks to all the employees and professionals of the Hospital for Rehabilitation of Craniofacial Anomalies, University of São Paulo (HRCA/USP), for their collaboration in clinical care and carrying out research projects. We also appreciate the collaboration of our friend Pricila Copedê Frascareli.

We also would like to thank our friends Henrique Regonaschi Serigatto *M.Sc.,* Juliana Mercado Santos *M.Sc.* and Dr Luiza do Amaral Virmond for collaborating with us on Chapters 17 and 18.

We wish to thank Elanor Harris for collaborating with proofreading this book.

We want to acknowledge *Coordenação de Aperfeiçoamento de Pessoal de Nível Superior* (PNPD/CAPES 88882.315687/2019-01 and AUXE/PROAP/

CAPES 14-2023 Programa de Pós-Graduação em Ciências da Reabilitação – 33002010182P0) by financial support.

INTRODUCTORY NOTE

Craniofacial clefts are uncommon congenital anomalies that affect facial bones and soft tissue structures, resulting in anatomical deficiencies (Tessier, 1976, David, Moore and Cooter, 1989). The exact frequency of rare craniofacial clefts is unknown. The estimated incidences of rare orofacial clefts have been reported as 1.43 to 4.85 per 100,000 live births (Kawamoto, 1976, Fijałkowska and Antoszewski, 2015).

Patients presenting some type of craniofacial cleft frequently need an extensive follow-up by a multidisciplinary team and different treatment protocols according to the type and amplitude of the cleft. The first author that recognized the three-dimensional complexity of cleft was Paul Tessier (1976), who established that a cleft in the soft tissue corresponds to a cleft in the bone structure. The Tessier classification (1976) consists of a numerical classification of the anatomical structures, considering the location of the cleft, taking the sagittal midline as a reference, both for soft and bone tissue. The orbit is the primary reference structure, and 15 regions are defined counter-clockwise. The clefts affecting the middle and upper craniofacial region are numbered from 0 to 14, and the mandibular cleft (lower face region) is 30 (Figure 1). Another classification was proposed for craniofacial clefts (van der Meulen, 1983). However, the Tessier classification is the most used. This study aims to morphologically evaluate the craniofacial structures involved in individuals with isolated or syndromic rare craniofacial clefts; to evaluate the association of bone and soft tissue clefts; and to contribute to the diagnosis, management and understanding of the pathogenetic mechanisms of these types of clefts. The computed tomography images of every patient were digitized and processed using the Mimics 17.0 software (Mimics, Materialize, Belgium). A craniofacial surgeon assisted the team in evaluating the computed tomography scans, and the orthodontists supervised the segmentation of craniofacial structures and the evaluation of craniofacial growth. This project was approved by the Research Ethics Committee (CEP-HRAC number 2.146.750/2017). The participants or legal guardians authorized all images and files from patients' photographs and computed tomography.

References

David, D. J., M. H. Moore, and R. D. Cooter. 1989. "Tessier Clefts Revisited with a Third Dimension." Cleft Palate J 26 (3): 184–85.

Fijałkowska, M., and B. Antoszewski. 2015. "Rare Facial Clefts." Pol Przegl Chir 87 (8): 389–94. https://doi.org/ 10.1515/pjs-2015-0077

Kawamoto, H. K. 1976. "The Kaleidoscopic World of Rare Craniofacial Clefts: Order out of Chaos (Tessier Classification)." Clin Plast Surg 3 (4): 529–72.

Meulen, J. C. van der, R. Mazzola, C. Vermey-Keers, M. Strieker, and B. Raphael. 1983. "A Morphogenetic Classification of Craniofacial Malformations." Plastic and Reconstructive Surgery 71 (4): 560–72. https://doi.org/10.1097/00006534-198304000-00022.

Tessier, Paul. 1976. "Anatomical Classification of Facial, Cranio-Facial and Latero-Facial Clefts." *Journal of Maxillofacial Surgery* 4: 69–92. https://doi.org/10.1016/s0301-0503(76)80013-6.

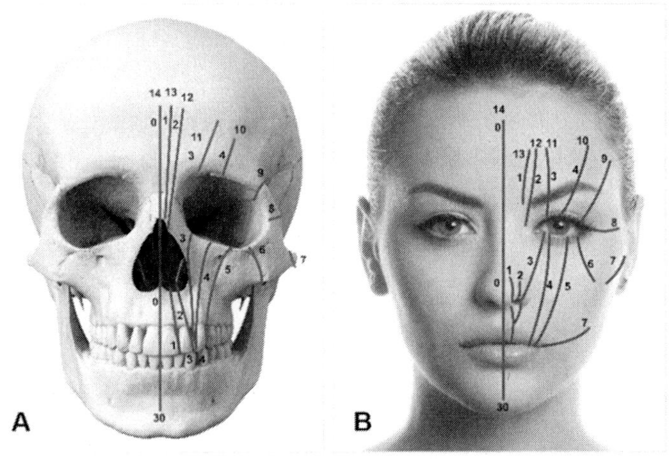

Figure 1 – Classification of the craniofacial clefts according to Tessier (1976). (A) Bone clefts numbered. (B) Soft tissue clefts numbered. Original artwork by the authors.

CHAPTER ONE

TESSIER CLEFT NUMBER 0: THE MEDIAN CLEFT LIP

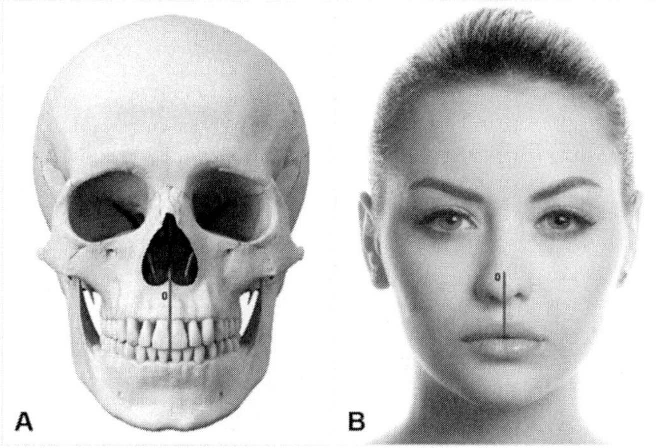

Figure 2 – Localization of Tessier cleft number 0. (A) Bone clefts numbered. (B) Soft tissue clefts numbered. Original artwork by the authors.

Tessier cleft number 0, also known as median cleft, is caused by the lack of fusion of the frontonasal and medial nasal processes. It can result in premaxilla agenesis (Figure 2). Cleft number 0 involves structures of the facial midline showing wide phenotypic variability and microforms. In some cases, the premaxilla may be partially affected. The cleft may present as a small notch in the upper lip, vermilion, or the alveolar arch (between the maxillary central incisors), with a bifid nose or a midline groove along the nasal dorsum. Tessier cleft number 0 can be associated with other midline anomalies, including hypotelorism or hypertelorism, holoprosencephaly, corpus callosum agenesis and frontonasal encephalocele. These combinations can be part of a known condition, such as holoprosencephaly (OMIM 236100), frontonasal dysplasia (OMIM 136760), orofacial digital syndrome (OMIM 311200), Pai syndrome

(155145), Sakoda complex (midline cleft, ethmoidal encephalocele, ocular anomaly, corpus callosum agenesis and cleft palate) (OMIM 610871), among others.

References

Baek, Seung-Hak, Yoon-Hee Park, Jee Hyeok Chung, Sukwha Kim, and Jin-Young Choi. 2018. "Orthodontic and Orthopedic Treatment for a Growing Patient with Tessier Number 0 Cleft." *Korean Journal of Orthodontics* 48 (2): 113–24. https://doi.org/10.4041/kjod.2018.48.2.113.

Cohen Jr MM. *Perspectives on the face*. Oxford University Press: New York; 2006

David, D. J., M. H. Moore, and R. D. Cooter. 1989. "Tessier Clefts Revisited with a Third Dimension." *Cleft Palate J* 26 (3): 184–85.

De Boutray, M., J. L. Beziat, J. Yachouh, M. Bigorre, A. Gleizal, and G. Captier. 2016. "Median Cleft of the Upper Lip: A New Classification to Guide Treatment Decisions." *J Craniomaxillofac Surg* 44 (6): 664–71.

Evans, Kelly N., Anne V. Hing, and Michael L. Cunningham. 2018. "Craniofacial Malformations." In *Avery's Diseases of the Newborn*, 1417-1437.e2. Elsevier.

Guruprasad, Y., and D. S. Chauhan. 2014. "Midline Nasal Dermoid Cyst with Tessier's 0 Cleft." *J Nat Sci Biol Med* 5 (2): 479–82.

Kolker, A. R., A. M. Sailon, J. G. Meara, and A. D. Holmes. 2015. "Midline Cleft Lip and Bifid Nose Deformity: Description, Classification and Treatment." *J Craniofac Surg* 26 (8): 2304–8.

Online Mendelian Inheritance in Man, OMIM®. McKusick-Nathans Institute of Genetic Medicine, Johns Hopkins University (Baltimore, MD). Accessed November 10, 2022. https://omim.org/.

Tessier, Paul. 1976. "Anatomical Classification of Facial, Cranio-Facial and Latero-Facial Clefts." *Journal of Maxillofacial Surgery* 4: 69–92. https://doi.org/10.1016/s0301-0503(76)80013-6.

Tessier cleft number 0

Case 1

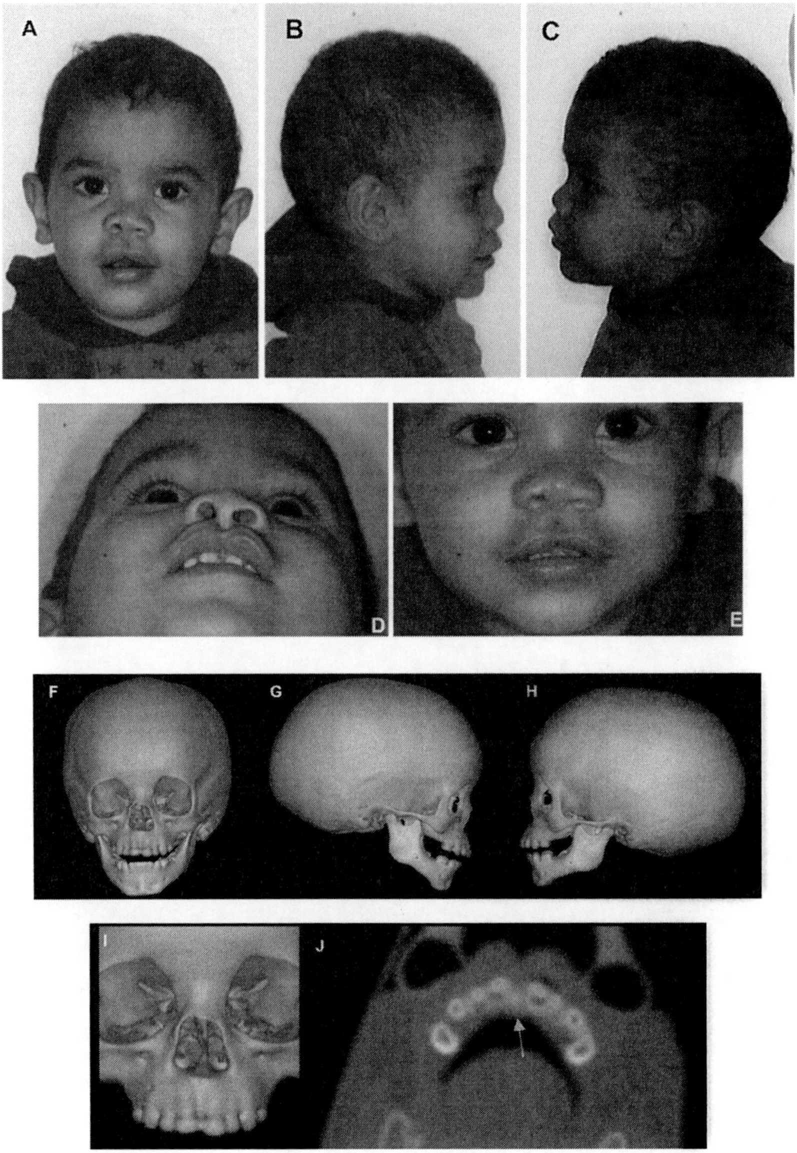

Figure 3 (previous page) – Clinical phenotype of a male patient with Tessier cleft number 0. A-E: Facial photographs at 12 months old. Note a mild midline cleft lip with separated vermillion and midline groove that extends until the philtrum. A wide nasal base with an asymmetrical nostril and a mild Tessier cleft number one (right side) on the nasal dorsum was presented with a furrow in the soft tissue. F-I: computed tomography 3D-reconstructions obtained at age 12 months (frontal, lateral and oblique view). I: observe a close mild alveolar cleft between the maxillary central incisors with a mild notch in the alveolar ridge. An asymmetrical nasal cavity with a mild notch in the left nasal bone was observed. J: computed tomography axial section showing a mild notch in the middle region of the maxillary alveolar ridge.

Case 2

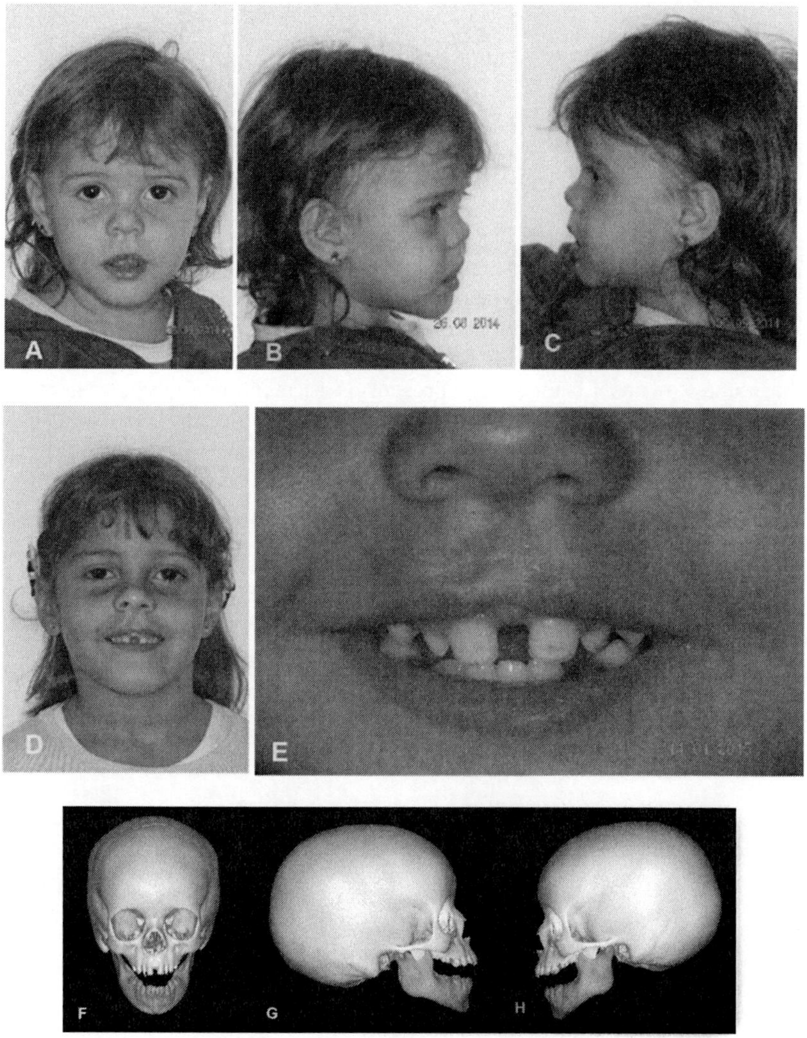

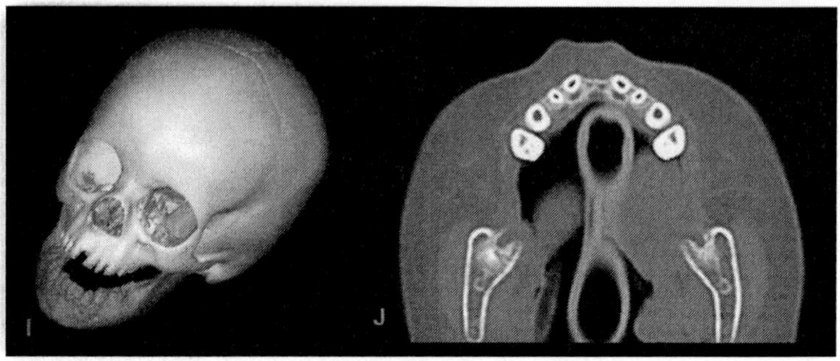

Figure 4 – Clinical phenotype of a female patient with Tessier cleft number 0. A-C: at one year and four months old. Observe the mild cleft at the centre of the upper lip extending as a wide groove in the philtrum. A wide nasal base and low nasal bridge were present. D-E: facial phenotype at age five showing a midline diastema between maxillary central incisors. F-I: computed tomography 3D-reconstructions obtained at two years old showing a mild midline groove in the premaxilla. J: computed tomography axial section showing a widened interdental bone septum between the maxillary central incisors.

Case 3

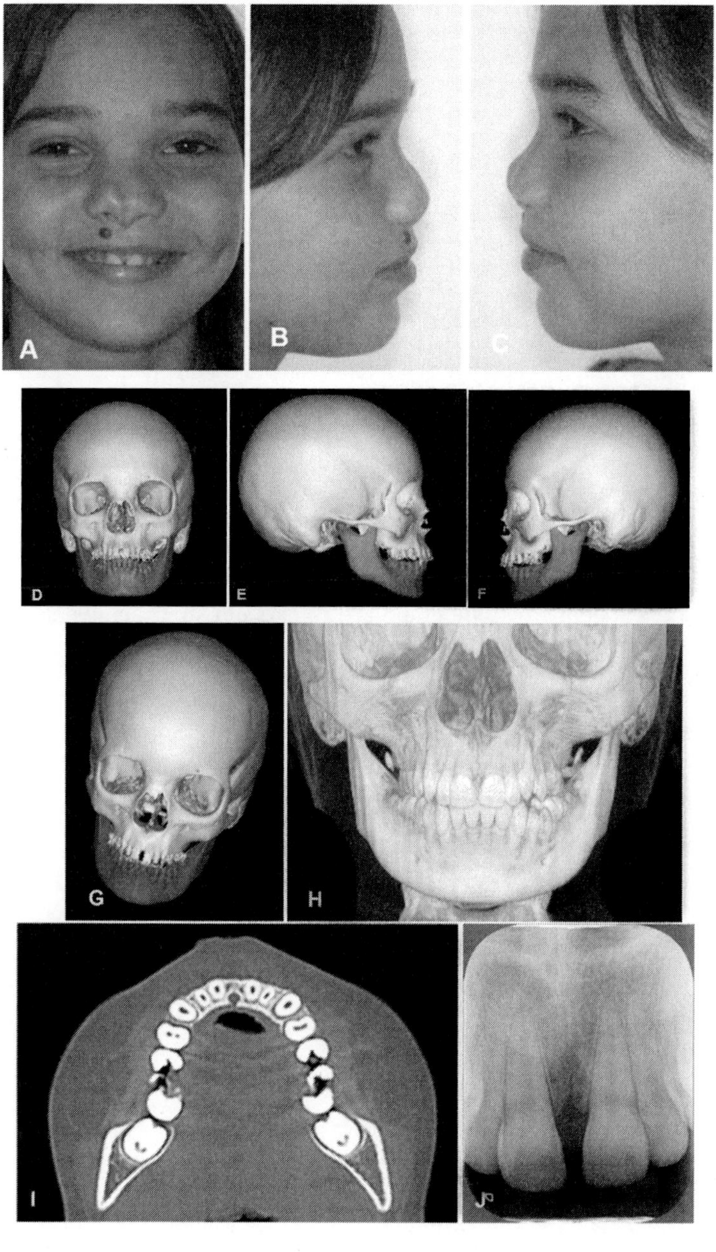

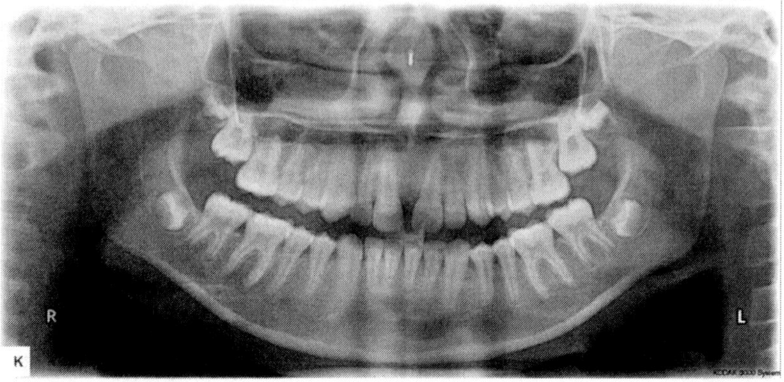

Figure 5 – Clinical phenotype of a ten-year-old female patient with Tessier cleft number 0. A-C: note the short nose with a wide and depressed nasal base, a large columella, a short philtrum and a nasal tip bifidity. D-G: computed tomography three-dimensional reconstruction obtained at ten years old. Observe a short and abnormal nasal bone and a midline diastema in the maxillary alveolar ridge. H-I: observe a small notch in the alveolar ridge between the central incisors. J: periapical radiography showing a V-shape midline bone defect in the alveolar ridge between the upper central incisors. K: panoramic radiograph at 11 years old showing alveolar defect between upper central incisors and absence of dental anomalies.

Case 4

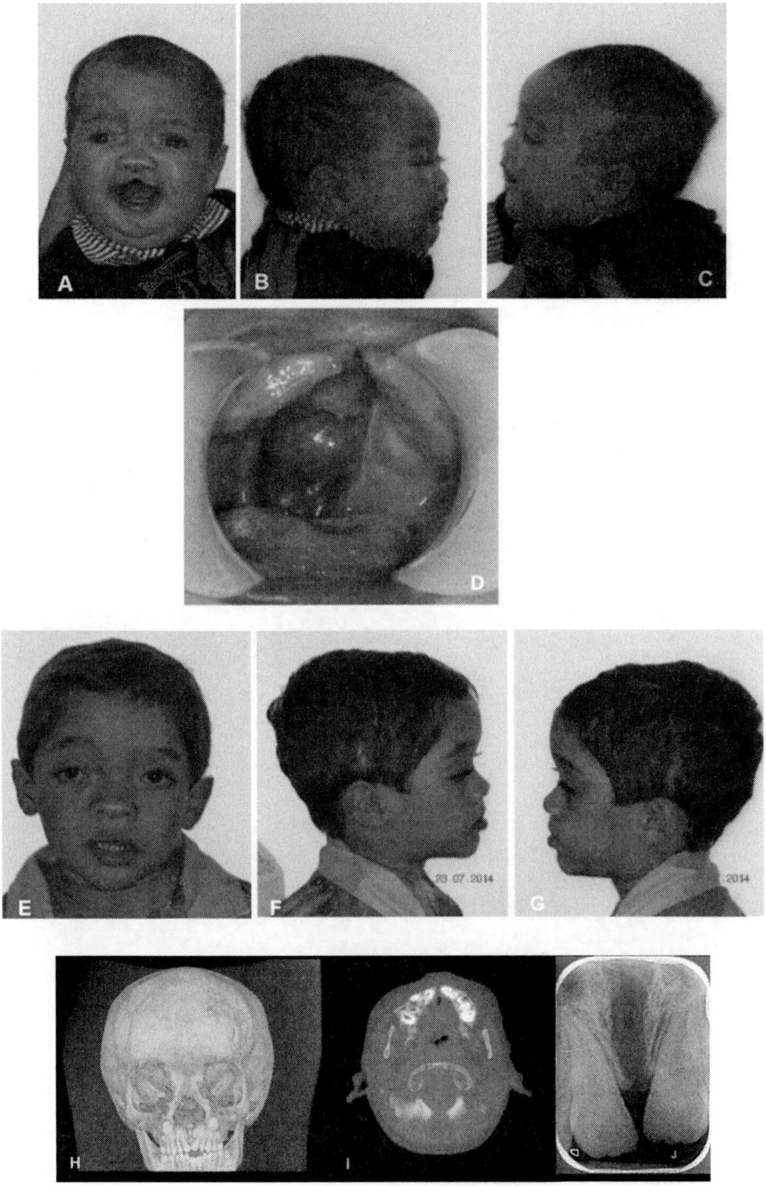

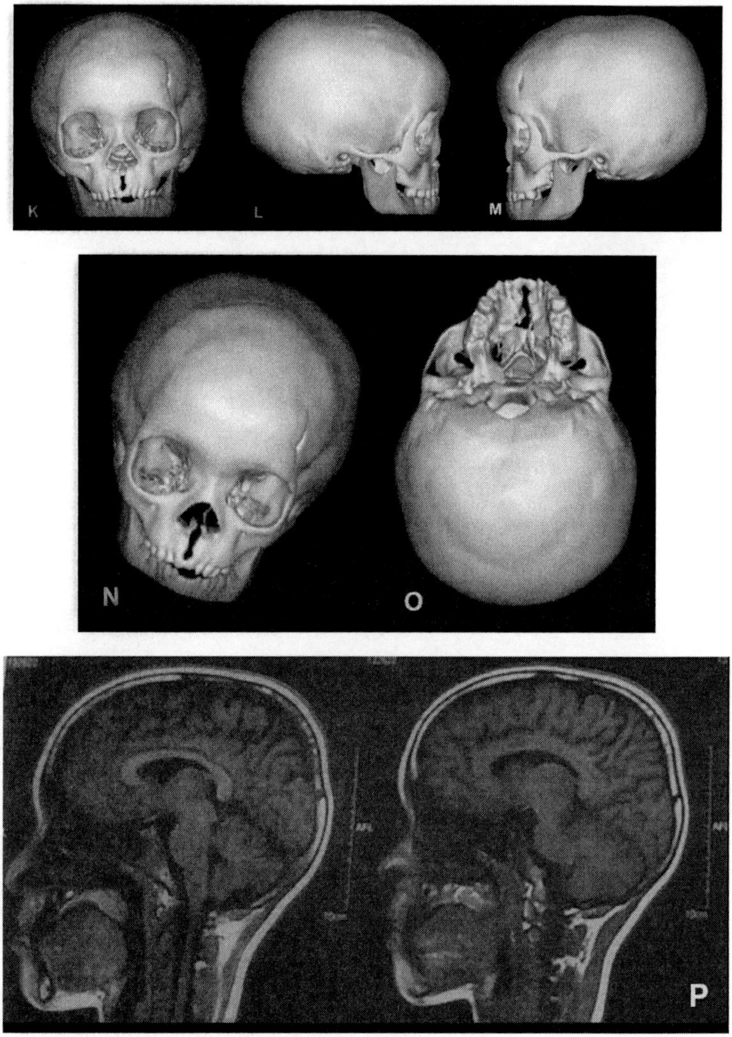
K
L
M
N
O
P

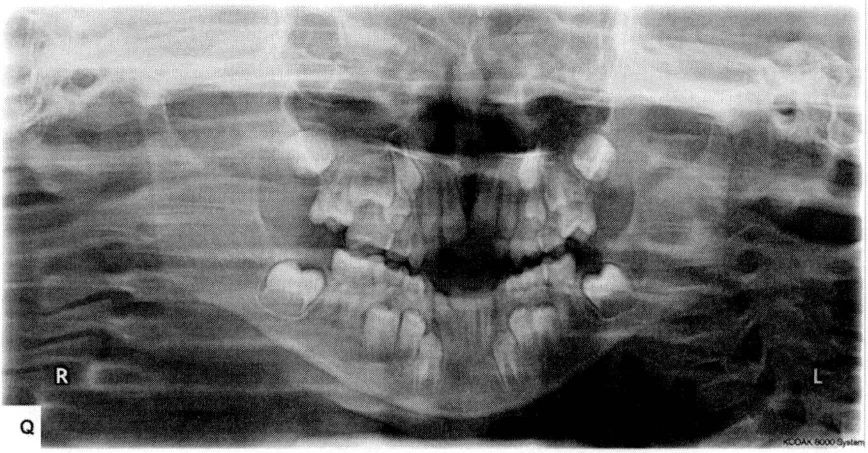

Figure 6 – Clinical phenotype of a male patient with Sakoda complex (OMIM 610871). A-D: at three months old, a short nose with a wide and depressed nasal base, large columella and midline cleft lip extending through vermillion and philtrum were observed. A midline cleft palate and basal cephalocele were present in the oral cavity. E-G: postoperative follow-up at five years old. Note the orbital hypertelorism and the wide nasal bridge. H: translucent computed tomography 3D reconstruction showing a maxillary midline cleft extending until the nasal cavity. I: computed tomography axial section showing a bone defect between the maxillary central incisors. J: periapical radiography showing a wide midline defect in the alveolar ridge between the maxillary central incisors. K-O: computed tomography 3D images obtained at five years old.

The midline cleft lip and palate were present. Observe the flat nasal bone, a vomer duplication, nasal septum deviation to the left, and (O) orthogonal occlusal view of the hard palate. P: magnetic resonance imaging at 12 years old showing brain structures. Q: panoramic radiograph at seven years old shows the alveolar defect between the upper central incisors and an absence of dental anomalies.

Case 5

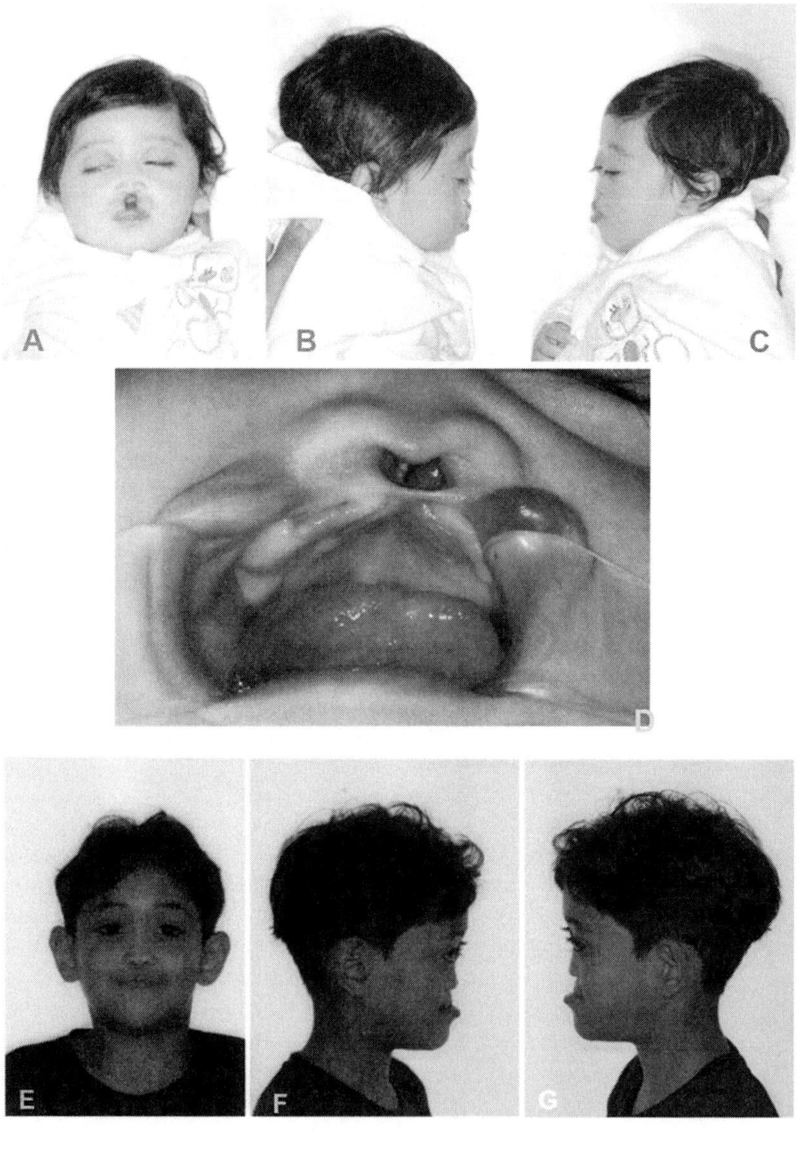

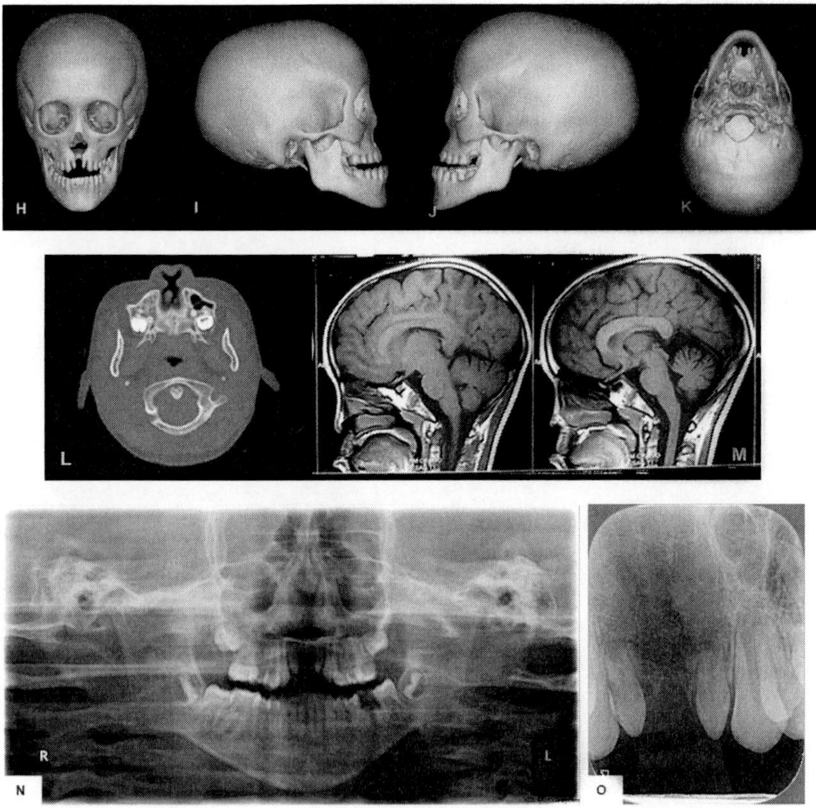

Figure 7 – Clinical phenotype of a male patient with holoprosencephaly-like. The facial phenotype is similar to holoprosencephaly except for the absence of an abnormal central nervous system. A-D: at three months old, note an ocular hypotelorism and a flat face with midface hypoplasia, depressed nasal base, absence of the nasal bridge, unique nasal cavity, absence of the columella and philtrum, a wide median cleft lip, and premaxilla agenesis with a V-shape defect in the central region of the maxillary alveolar arch. E-G: postoperative follow-up at nine years old. Observe the orbital hypertelorism and midface hypoplasia with a flat nasal bridge. H-J: computed tomography 3D-reconstructions obtained at nine years old. Note the lateral displacement of the nasal processes of the maxilla, the absence of the vomer and anterior nasal spine, and the absence of premaxilla with a wide midline cleft. Small lateral incisors were present in the mesial region of the maxillary processes. K: bottom view of CT 3D

reconstruction showing the median cleft restricted to the alveolar arch with a normal hard palate. L: computed tomography axial section showing the absence of the nasal septum. M: magnetic resonance imaging at nine years old shows midface hypoplasia, premaxilla agenesis and a normal central nervous system. N: panoramic radiograph at nine years old showing central maxillary defect with the upper central incisors agenesis. O: periapical radiography showing the maxillary defect and bilateral conoid tooth (lateral incisors maxillary).

Case 6

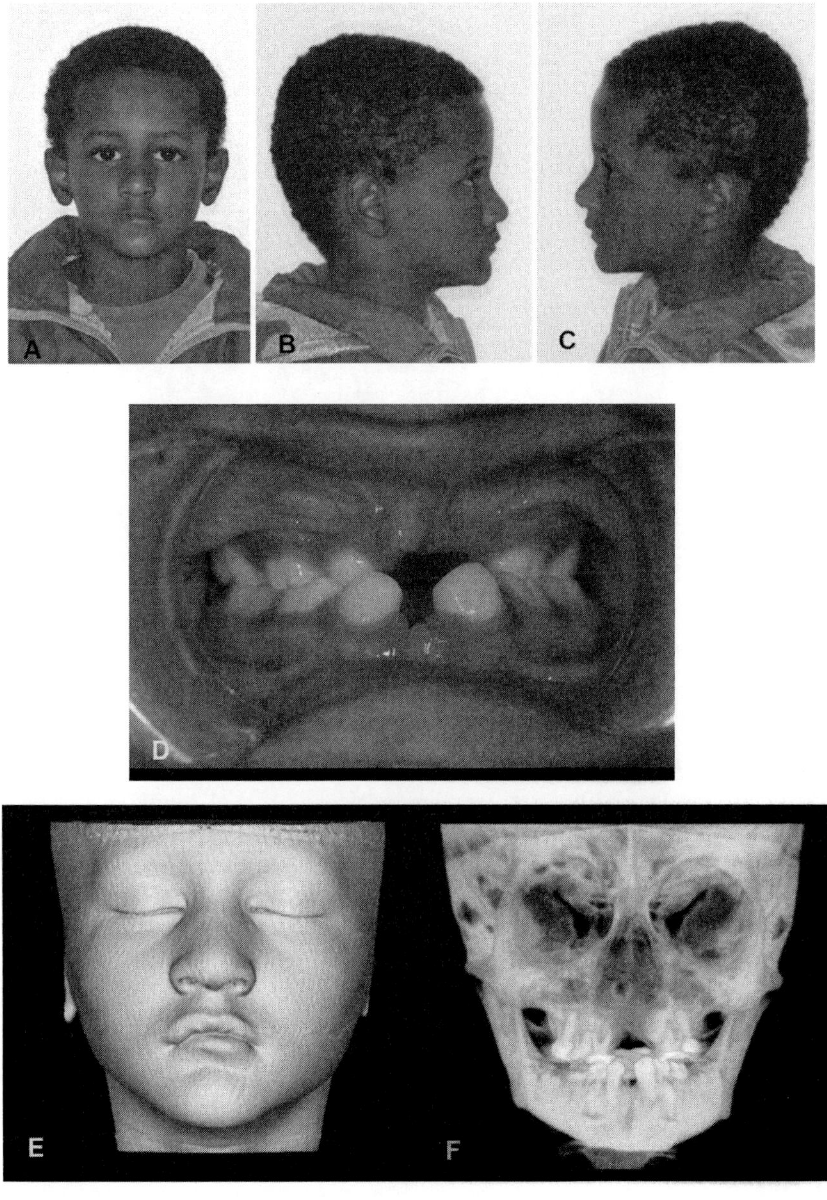

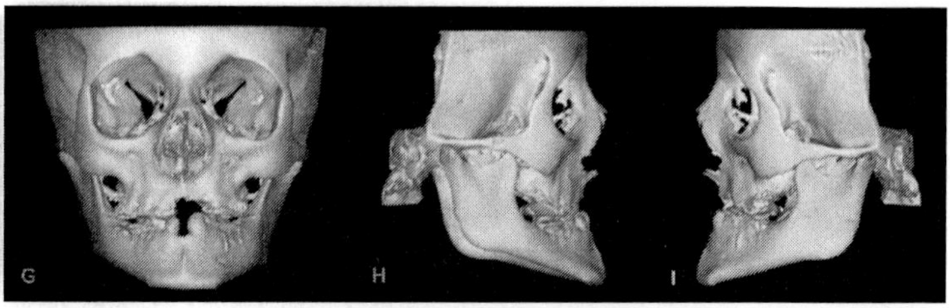

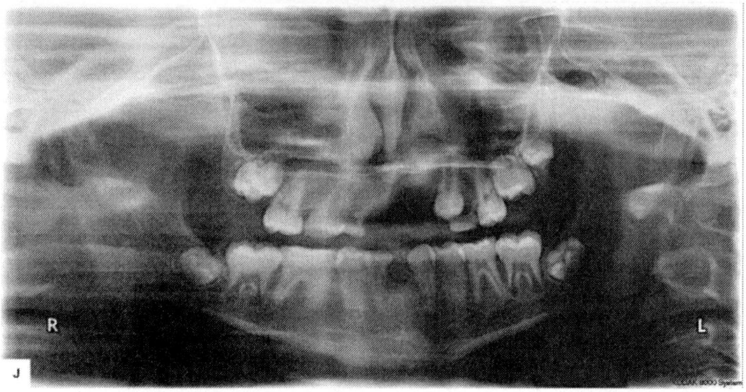

Figure 8 – Clinical phenotype of a male patient with hypoglossia. A-D: At seven years old, note a mild facial asymmetry in the mandibular region in the soft tissue. A mild alveolar midline defect with the absence of the maxillary central and lateral incisors (Tessier cleft number 0) and the absence of the first premolar and canine bilaterally, a mandibular midline alveolar cleft (Tessier cleft number 30) with the absence of mandibular central and lateral incisors, first premolar at right and canine at left. E-I: computed tomography 3D images obtained at 11 years old. Figure E shows no soft tissue clefts. Only an asymmetry was observed in the lower lip and the mandibular region. The translucent CT reconstruction (Figure F) confirmed the premaxilla agenesis and a mandibular alveolar cleft. In frontal and lateral views of the cranium (Figures G to I), observe the midface hypoplasia and mild midline cleft (Tessier bone cleft number 0) extending to the premaxilla as a groove. Note a midline mandibular cleft (Tessier number 30). J: panoramic radiograph at 14 years old showing central alveolar defects in maxilla and mandible and multiple dental agenesis (14, 13, 12, 11, 21, 22, 23, 24, 32, 33, 31, 41, 42, 44).

Case 7

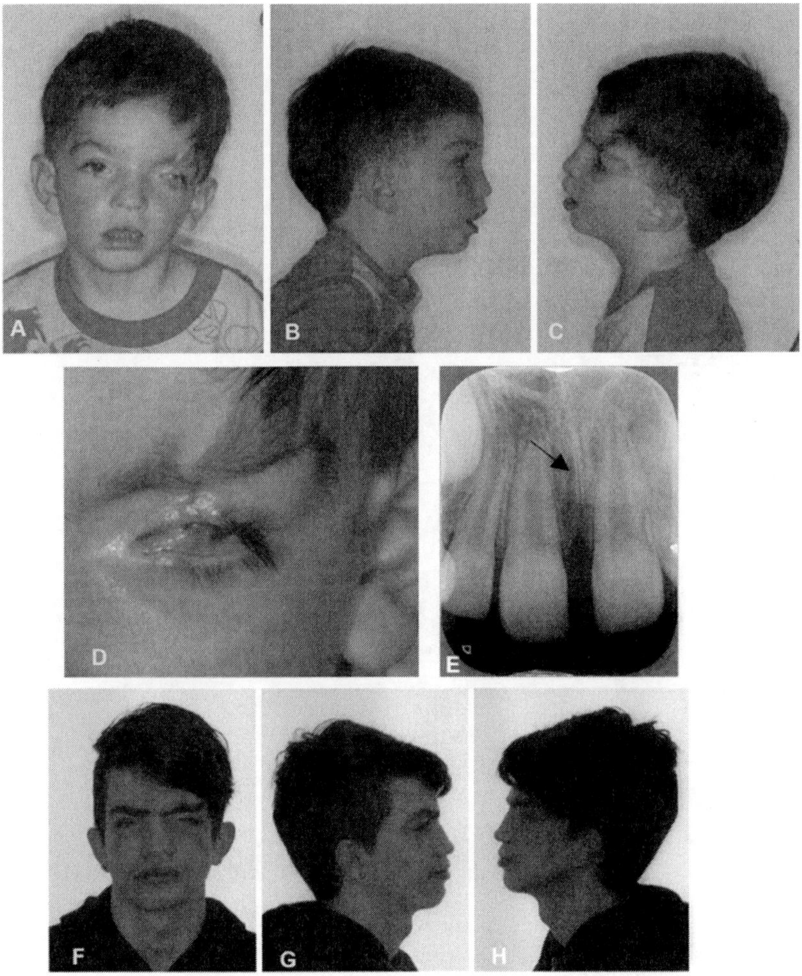

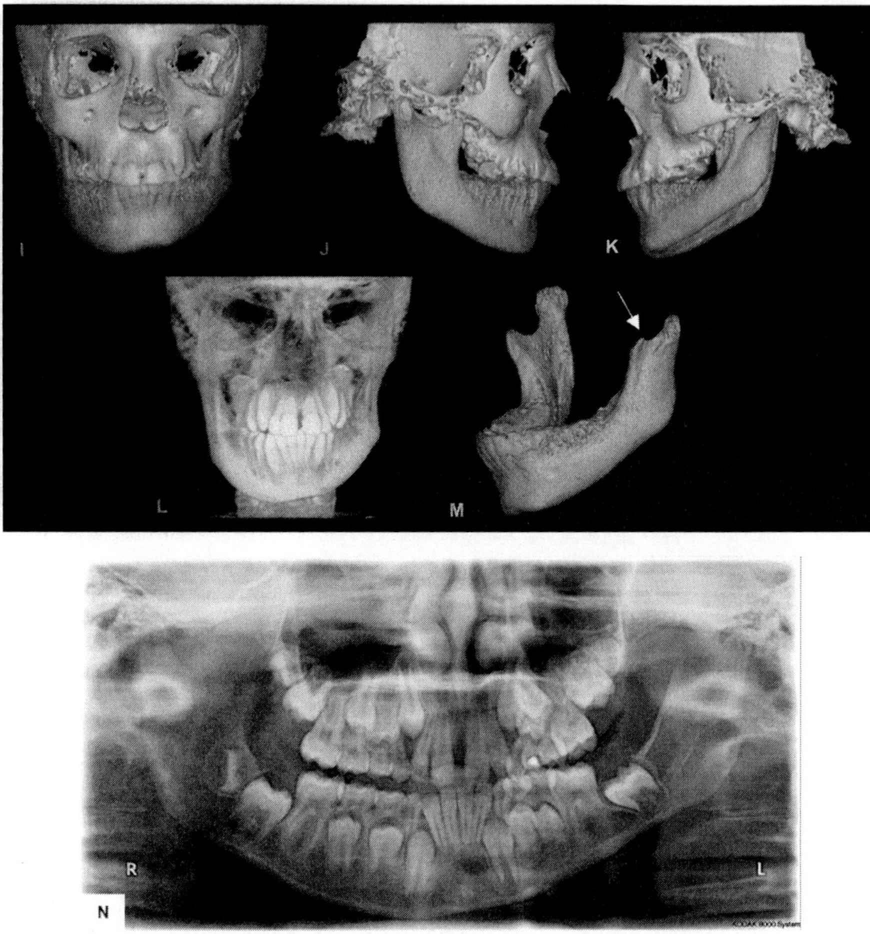

Figure 9 – Clinical phenotype of a male patient with oculoauriculofrontonasal syndrome (OMIM 601452). A-D: At three years old, note a slight facial asymmetry and an ocular abnormality on the left side in the soft tissue. In Figure D, the left eye demonstrated an abnormal upper palpebral fissure with an irregular upper eyelid and eyelashes extending to the middle region of the eyebrow (Tessier cleft number 11). E: periapical radiography showing a midline defect in the alveolar ridge between the maxillary central incisors. F-H: facial phenotype at 14 years old. I-K: computed tomography 3D-reconstructions obtained at age 12 showing a mandibular asymmetry and a midline notch in the maxillary

alveolar arch (Tessier cleft number 0). L: computed tomography translucent 3D- reconstruction showing a mild midline defect between the maxillary central incisors. M: mandibular 3D reconstruction revealing a condyle and coronoid process hypoplasia on the left side (arrow shows the left side). N: panoramic radiograph at ten years old showing the upper central alveolar defect and absence of dental anomalies.

CHAPTER TWO

TESSIER CLEFT NUMBER 1: THE PARAMEDIAN CLEFT

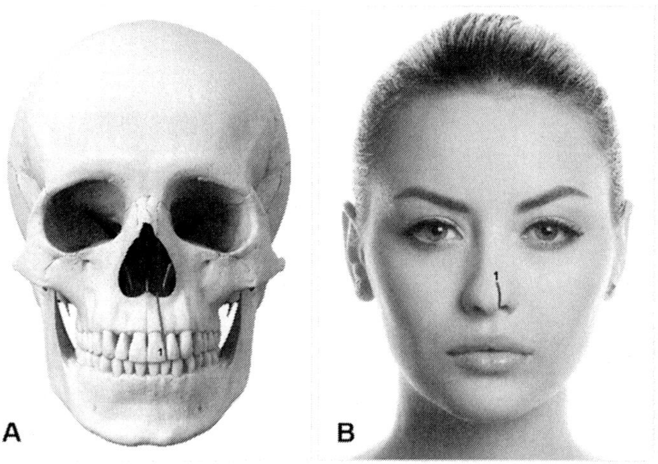

Figure 10 – Localization of Tessier cleft number 1. (A) Bone clefts numbered. (B) Soft tissue clefts numbered. Original artwork by the authors.

Tessier cleft number 1 is similar to the typical cleft lip and palate but extends to the alae nasi. The Tessier cleft number 1 occurs due to a developmental abnormality in the frontonasal process, consequently lacking fusion between the nasomedial and nasolateral processes. It is characterized by a cleft in the nasal wing (or alae nasi) while the septum remains preserved (Figure 10). The phenotype can vary from a notch to the absence of the nostril wings and involvement of the nasal bone. Ocular hypertelorism might occur when the cleft reaches the ethmoid region. In these cases, the cleft extends to the cephalic region between the lateral nasal bone and the frontal process of the maxilla. At the level of bone tissue, the Tessier cleft number 1 can affect the alveolar region between the central and lateral incisors and the lateral wall of the pyriform aperture.

References

Aldabaany, Waleed. 2021. "Reconstruction of Congenital Alar Rim Defects (Tessier Number 1 Cleft) Using Laterally Based Alar Subunit Rotation Advancement Flap." *Annals of Plastic Surgery* 87 (2): 161–64. https://doi.org/10.1097/sap.0000000000002670.

David, D. J., M. H. Moore, and R. D. Cooter. 1989. "Tessier Clefts Revisited with a Third Dimension." *Cleft Palate J* 26 (3): 184–85.

Losee, J. E., R. E. Kirschner, L. A. Whitaker, and S. P. Bartlett. 2004. "Congenital Nasal Anomalies: A Classification Scheme." *Plast Reconstr Surg* 113 (2): 676–89. https://doi.org/10.1097/01.PRS.0000101540.32533.EC.

Ortiz Monasterio, F. 1987. "Fuente Del Campo A, Dimopulos A. Nasal Clefts." Ann Plast Surg 18 (5): 377–97.

Shewmake, K. B., and H. K. Kawamoto. 1992. "Congenital Clefts of the Nose: Principles of Surgical Management." Cleft Palate Craniofac J 29 (6): 531–39.

Stupka, Walther. 1950. "The Etiology of Lateral Nasal Clefts." Am J Pathol 26 (6):1085-1095.

Tessier, Paul. 1976. "Anatomical Classification of Facial, Cranio-Facial and Latero-Facial Clefts." Journal of Maxillofacial Surgery 4: 69–92. https://doi.org/10.1016/s0301-0503(76)80013-6.

Vesnel, S. L., and E. B. Wolvius. 2011. "Long-Term Results after 40 Years' Experience with Treatment of Rare Facial Clefts: Part 1-Oblique and Paramedian Clefts." J Plast Reconstr Aesthet Surg 64 (10): 1334–43. https://doi.org/10.1016/j.bjps.2011.04.021.

Winters, Ryan. 2016. "Tessier Clefts and Hypertelorism". *Facial Plastic Surgery Clinics of North America* 24 (4): 545–58. https://doi.org/10.1016/j.fsc.2016.06.013.

Tessier cleft number 1

Case 8

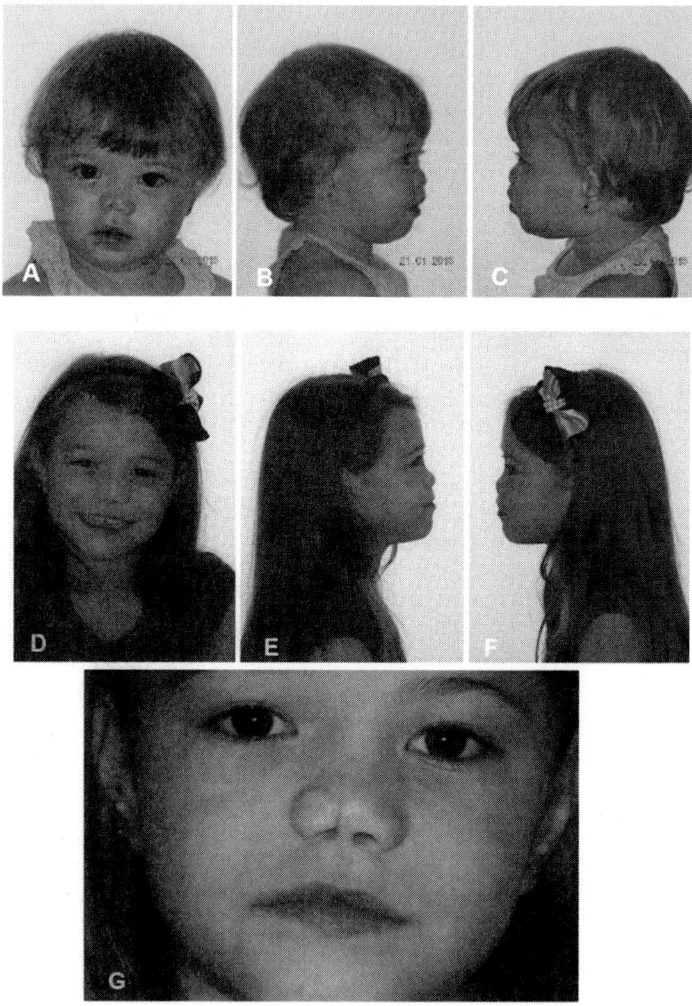

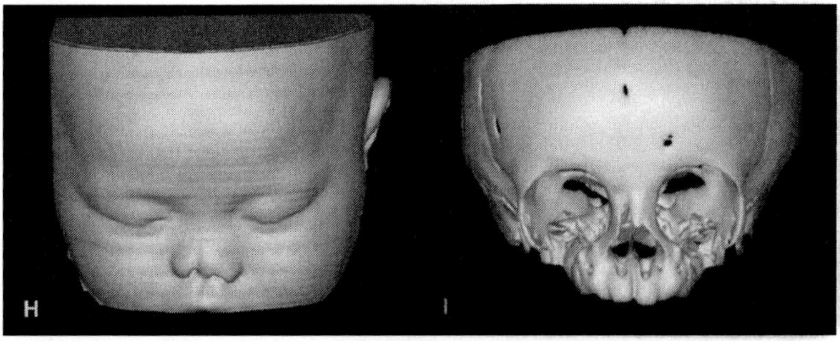

Figure 11– Clinical phenotype of a female patient with Tessier cleft number 1. A-C: at one year old, the base and nasal bridge were depressed with a paramedian cleft on the right nostril, abnormal nasal tip and short columella with deviation to the left side. A midline cleft was observed in the upper lip (Tessier cleft number 0). D-G: facial photographs at six years old. Observe the midline cleft lip with separated vermillion. H-I: computed tomography 3D reconstruction obtained at nine months old. In Figure H, observe that the alar cleft at the nose extended above the nasal dorsum as a paramedian cleft. In Figure I, a defect in the nasal bone on the right (Tessier cleft number 1) and a notch between the maxillary central incisor extending to the premaxilla (Tessier cleft number 0) were observed.

Case 9

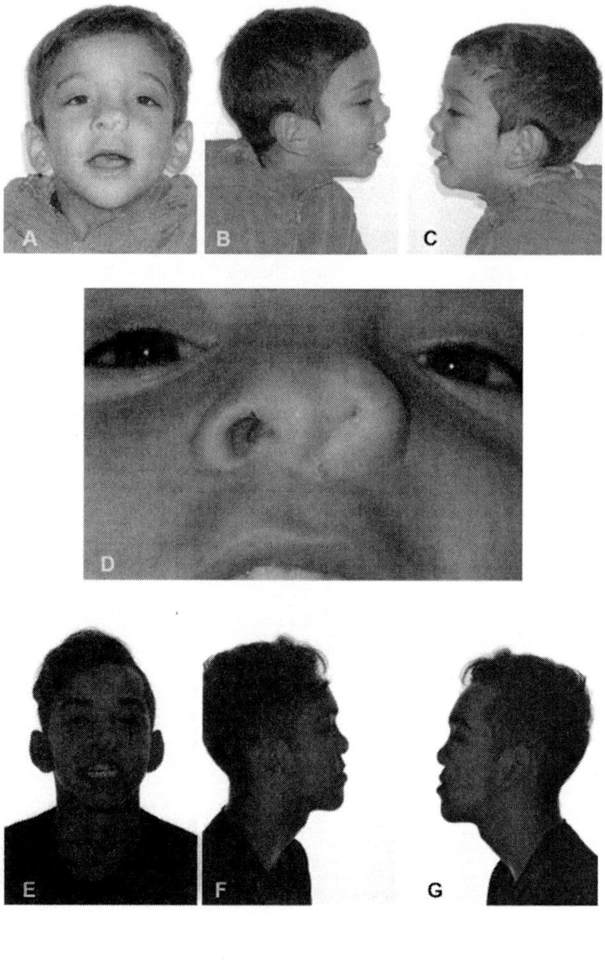

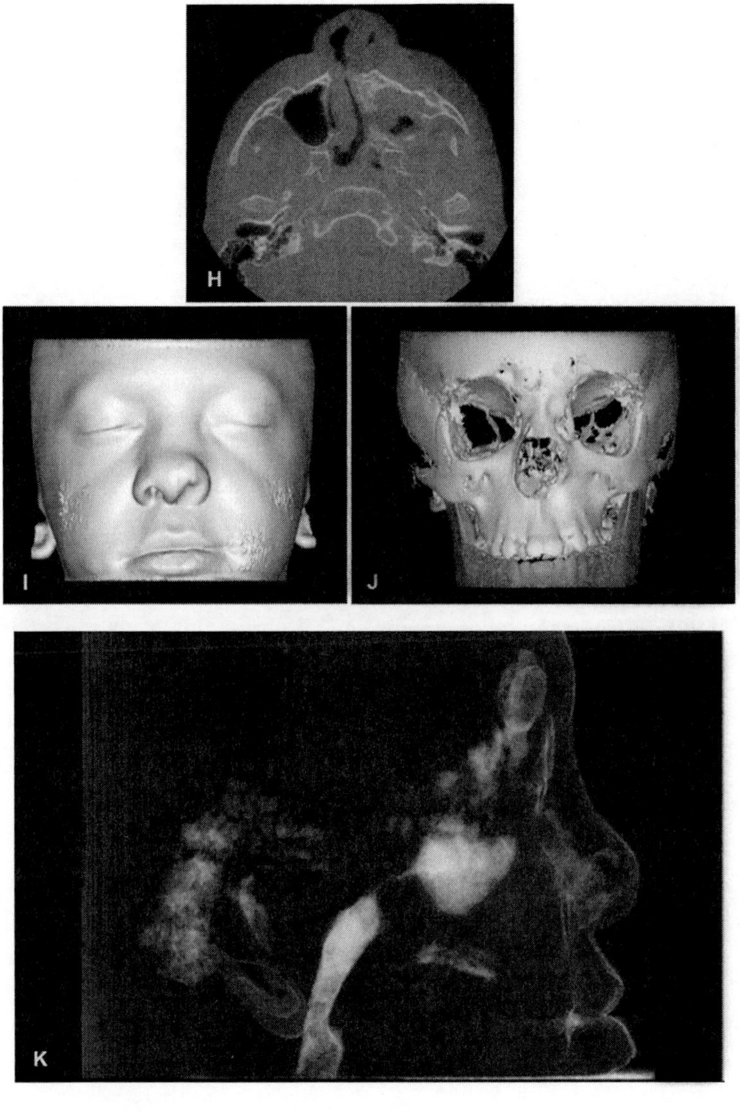
H
I
J
K

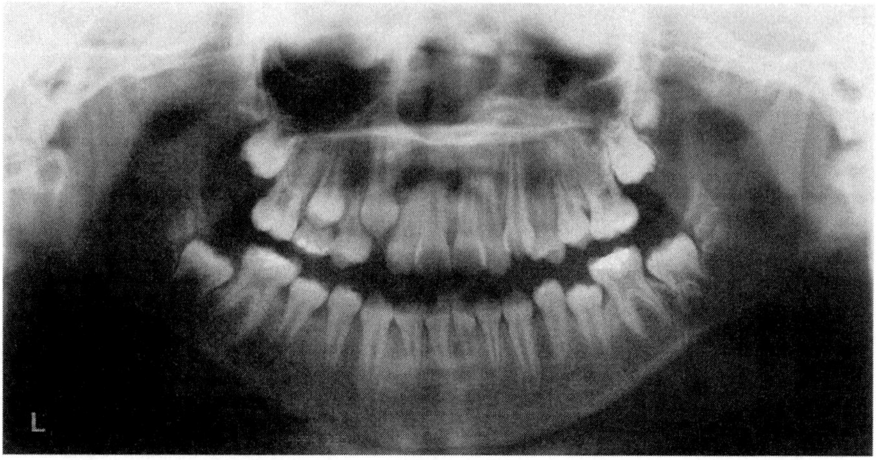

Figure 12 – Clinical phenotype of a male patient with Tessier cleft number 1. A-D: at five years old, observe the wide nasal base and bridge, the depressed nasal base on the left side, a paramedian cleft on the left side and a narrow nostril left. Figure D demonstrates hypoplasia of the columella and nasal tip. E-G: facial photographs at 15 years old. Note the midface hypoplasia. H: computed tomography axial section showing a malformation of the nasal cavity, septum and left maxillary sinus. I-J: computed tomography 3D-reconstructions obtained at 13 years old. A left paramedian cleft in the soft tissue is associated with a bone curvature of the nasal floor on the same side. (K) lateral view of the airway space. L: panoramic radiograph at ten years old shows no dental anomalies.

CHAPTER THREE

TESSIER CLEFT NUMBER 2: THE ALAR NASAL CLEFT

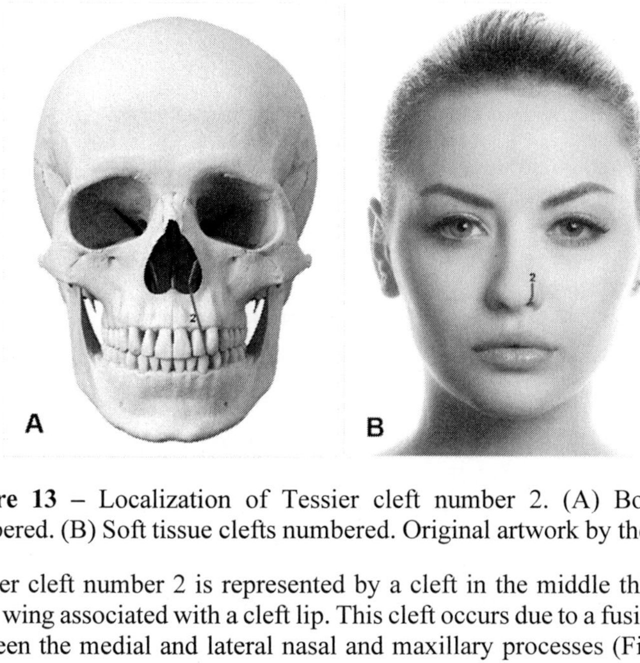

Figure 13 – Localization of Tessier cleft number 2. (A) Bone clefts numbered. (B) Soft tissue clefts numbered. Original artwork by the authors.

Tessier cleft number 2 is represented by a cleft in the middle third of the nasal wing associated with a cleft lip. This cleft occurs due to a fusion failure between the medial and lateral nasal and maxillary processes (Figure 13). The nasal alae are hypoplastic and might not have a real notch. In cases with a complete cleft, the nasal base and bridge are wide resulting in hypertelorism. At the soft tissue level, the cleft is represented by a deformity in the middle third of the edge of the nostril. At the bone tissue, the cleft begins at the maxillary alveolar ridge, extends into the pyriform cavity, and, in some cases, involves the nasal process of the maxilla superiorly.

References

Bütow, Kurt-W and Hanlie Engelbrecht. 2014. "Tessier 2 Nasal Cleft: Reconstruction with a Resorbable Sheet." *The British Journal of Oral & Maxillofacial Surgery* 52 (1): 93–94. https://doi.org/10.1016/j.bjoms.2013.05.148.

Chapchay, Katya, Jonathan Zaga, Allan Billig, Neta Adler and Alexander Margulis. 2019. "Surgical Technique for Nasal Cleft Repair." *Annals of Plastic Surgery* 82 (3): 289–91. https://doi.org/10.1097/SAP.0000000000001688.

David, D. J., M. H. Moore, and R. D. Cooter. 1989. "Tessier Clefts Revisited with a Third Dimension." *The Cleft Palate Journal* 26 (3): 163–84; discussion 184-5.

Guion-Almeida, Maria Leine and Antonio Richieri-Costa. 2010. "Frontonasal Dysgenesis, First Branchial Arch Anomalies, and Pericallosal Lipoma: A New Subtype of Frontonasal Dysgenesis." *American Journal of Medical Genetics. Part A* 152A (8): 2039–42. https://doi.org/10.1002/ajmg.a.33485.

Ortiz Monasterio, F. 1987. "Fuente Del Campo A, Dimopulos A. Nasal Clefts." *Ann Plast Surg* 18 (5): 377–97.

Monasterio, Fernando Ortiz, Antonio Fuente del Campo and Andres Dimopulos. 1987. "Nasal Clefts." *Annals of Plastic Surgery* 18 (5): 377. https://doi.org/10.1097/00000637-198705000-00004.

Ozek, Cuneyt, Hakan Gundogan, Ufuk Bilkay, Ruhi Cankayali, Ulvi Guner, Tahir Gurler and Ecmel Songur. 2001. "Rare Craniofacial Anomaly: Tessier No. 2 Cleft." *The Journal of Craniofacial Surgery* 12 (4): 355–61. https://doi.org/10.1097/00001665-200107000-00008.

Tessier, Paul. 1976. "Anatomical Classification of Facial, Cranio-Facial and Latero-Facial Clefts." *Journal of Maxillofacial Surgery* 4: 69–92. https://doi.org/10.1016/s0301-0503(76)80013-6.

Tiwari, P., S. K. Bhatnagar, and G. S. Kalra. 1991. "Tessier Number 2 Cleft, a Variation. Case Report." *Journal of Cranio-Maxillo-Facial Surgery: Official Publication of the European Association for Cranio-Maxillo-Facial Surgery* 19 (8): 346–47.

Tessier cleft number 2

Case 10

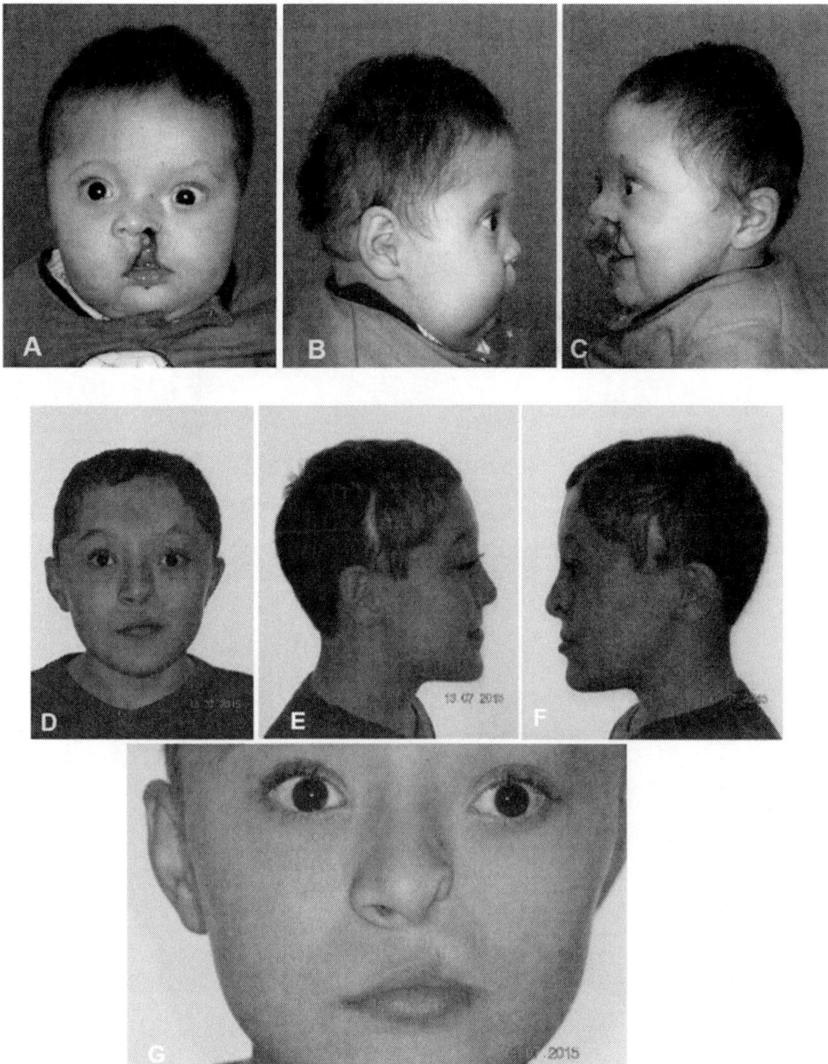

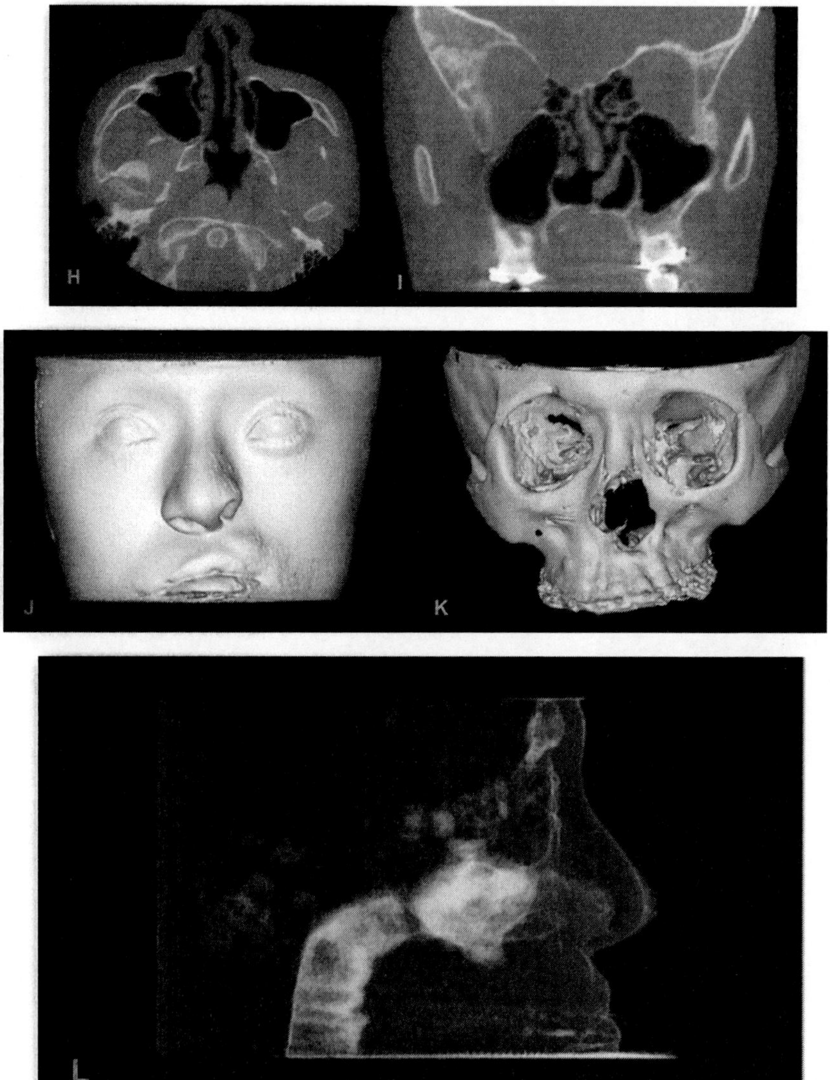
H
I
J
K
L

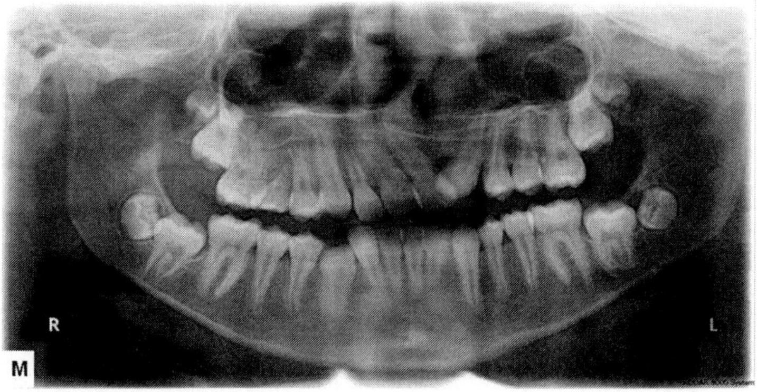

Figure 14 – Clinical phenotype of a male patient showing a Tessier cleft number 2. A-C: At seven months old, observe a wide cleft lip on the left side associated with a notch of the medial third of the nasal alae. D-G: facial photograph at age 11. A notch in the eyebrow on the left, midface hypoplasia and a slight asymmetry of the maxilla are observed. H–I: computed tomography axial and coronal sections obtained at 15 showed a malformation of the nasal cavity and a deviated nasal. J-K: computed tomography 3D-reconstructions reveal alae nasi cleft (Tessier cleft number 2) in soft tissue. An abnormal curvature of the nasal floor is observed at the bone tissue level. L: a normal upper airway is observed in the CT sagittal view. M: panoramic radiograph at 12 years old showing agenesis of the maxillary lateral incisor (22) and maxillary second premolar (15). Alveolar defects (between 21–23).

Case 11

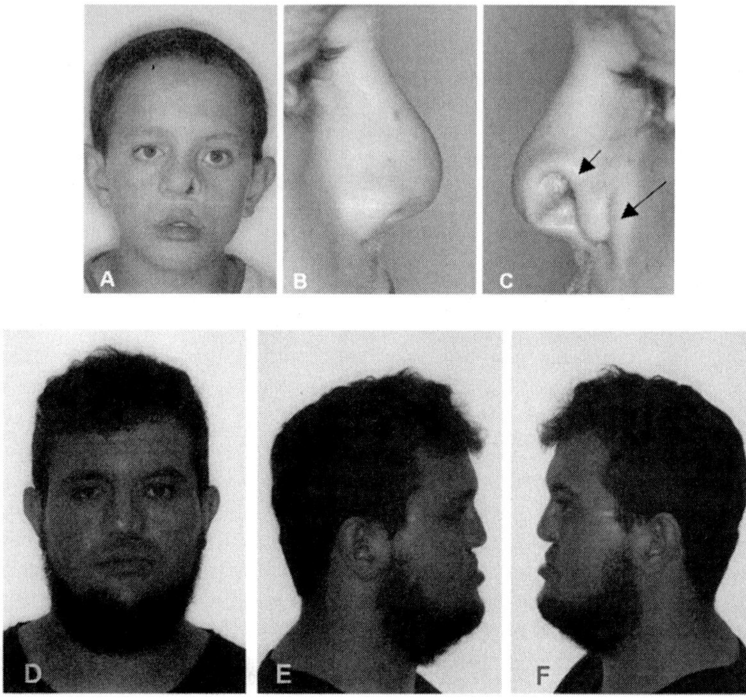

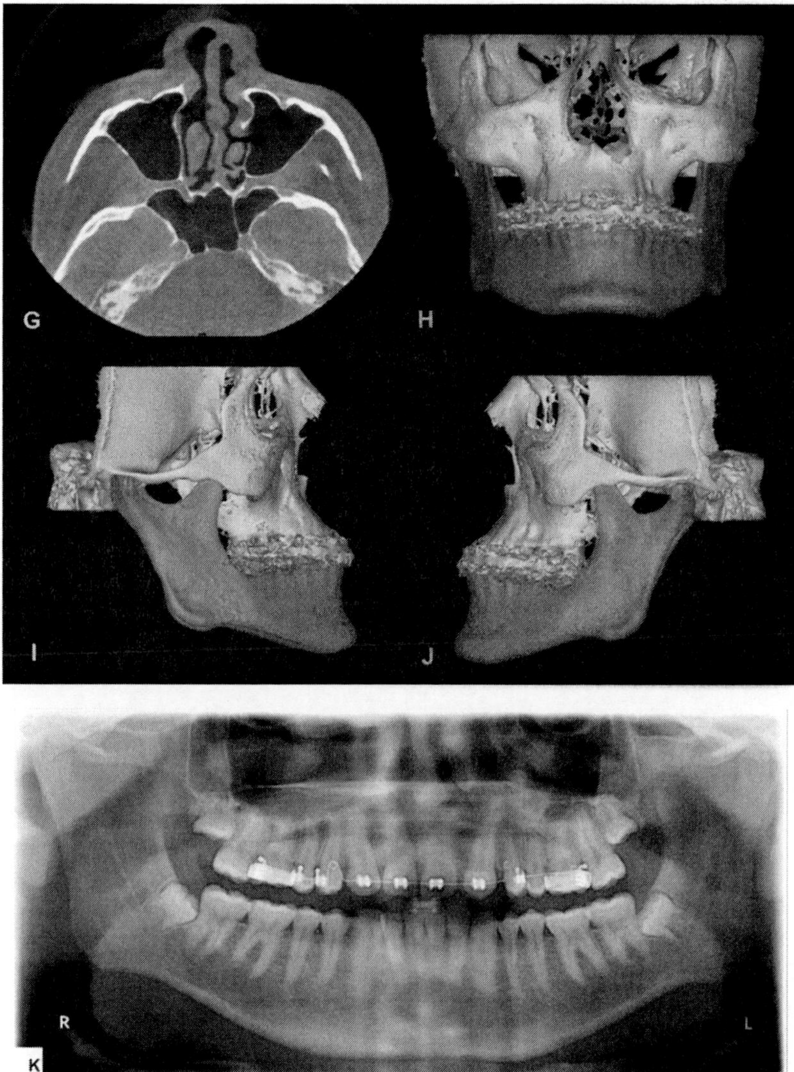

Figure 15 – Male patient showing a Tessier cleft number 2. A-C: at nine years old, note the alae nasi cleft in the nose (Tessier cleft number 2) on the left side, a repaired left cleft lip extending to the margin of the alae nasi (arrow), proceeding to the inner canthus of the lower eyelid as a mild groove (incomplete Tessier cleft number 3). D-F: facial phenotype at 21 years old.

The clefts were repaired, and a midface hypoplasia was observed. G: computed tomography axial section showing malformation of the nasal cavity with a deviated nasal septum. H-J: computed tomography 3D reconstructions obtained at age 21. Observe a paramedian cleft in the left maxilla, increasing the curvature of the nasal floor, midface hypoplasia and a relative mandibular protrusion. K: panoramic radiograph at 12 years old showing agenesis of the maxillary lateral incisor at left (22) and absence of a maxillary lateral incisor at right (12) (orthodontic extraction).

Case 12

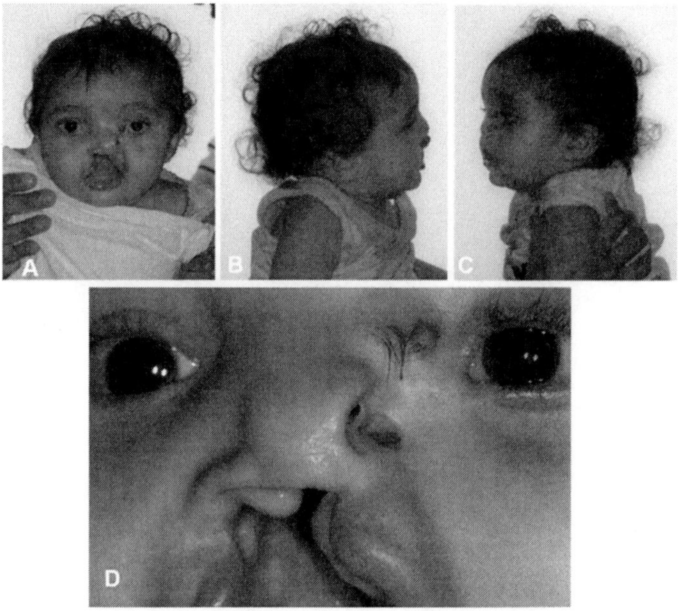

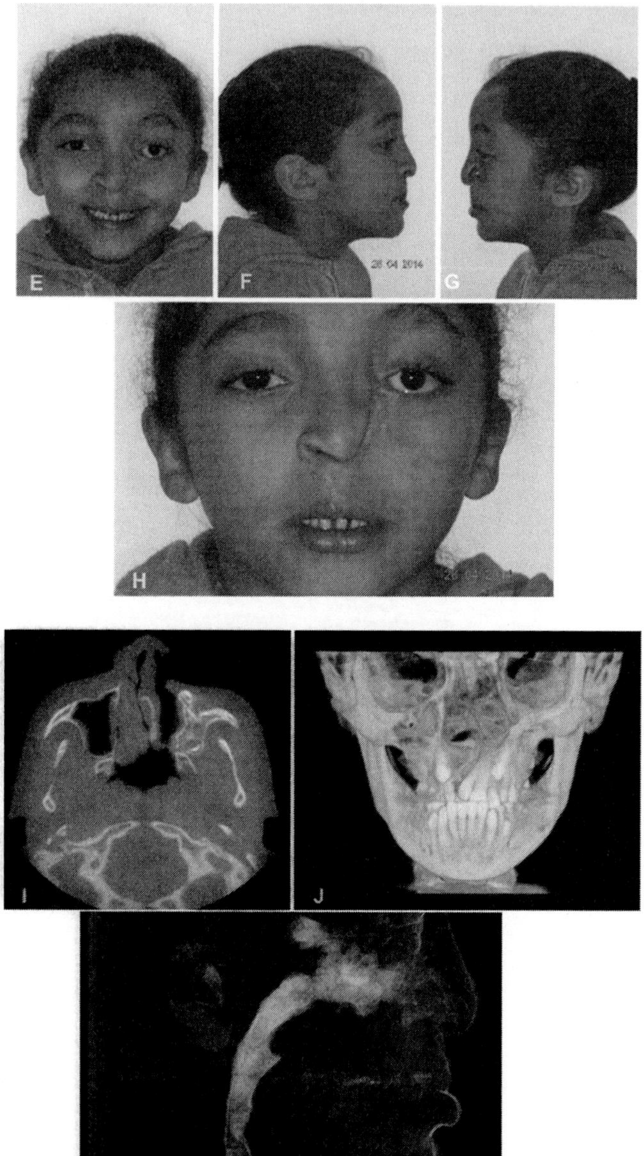
E
F
G
H
I
J
K

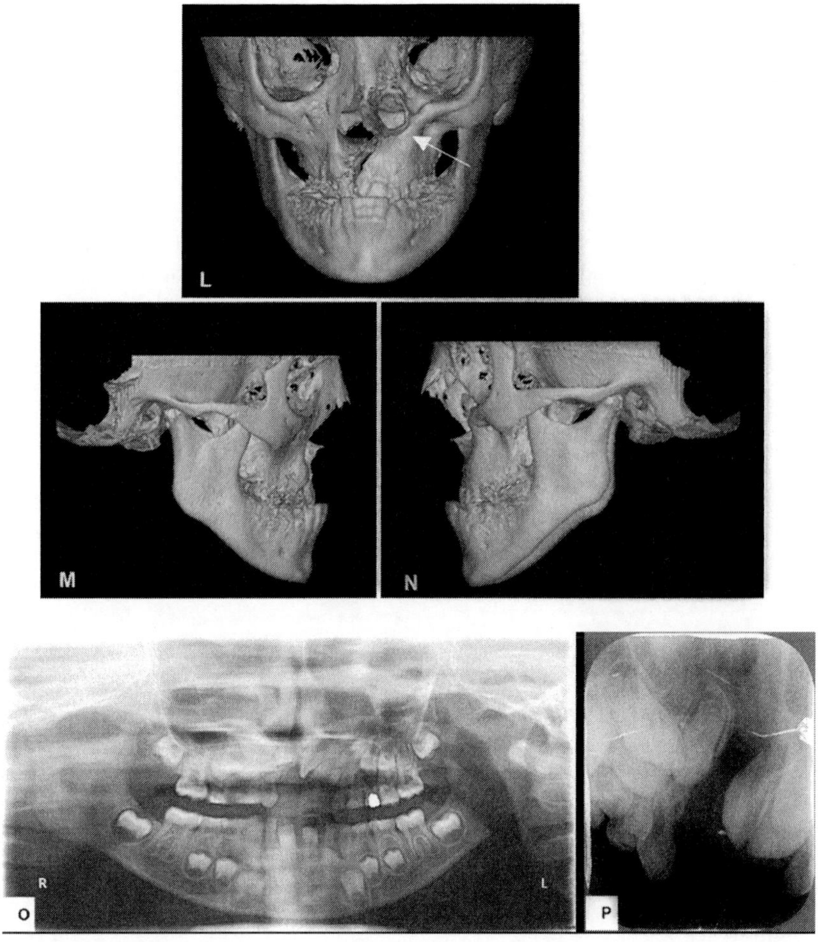

Figure 16 – Female patient with a Tessier cleft number 2. A-C: at six months old, observe the failure in the fusion between the medionasal and the maxillary processes on the left and right sides, ocular hypertelorism, an ectopic palpebral tissue with displacement eyelashes and a hypoplastic lacrimal puncta on the left side, the nasal root and bridge depression, the nasal tip with deviation to the right side, a wide cleft lip and palate on the right side with a deviation of the premaxilla to the left, a paramedian cleft on the left side (Tessier cleft number 2) with a wide pit in the nasolacrimal region and a groove extending inferiorly in the punctum lacrimal region. D: note the nasal asymmetry caused by the malpositioning of the nasal tip and

columella, a wide pit on the left side_and an atopic piliform tissue. E-G: facial photographs at seven years old with repaired cleft lip and nasal cleft. Observe the midface hypoplasia. I: computed tomography axial section showing the nasal septum deviated to the right. J: computed tomography 3D translucent reconstruction showing a wide and structurally abnormal nasal cavity. K: the upper airway in the lateral view was normal. L-N: computed tomography 3D reconstructions obtained at 11 years old. Observe the wide cleft lip and palate on the right side following a transversal line that crosses the nasal cavity and extends to the lateral middle third of the rim of the nostril on the left side and continues towards the left nasal bone, and the frontal process of the maxilla and inferior orbital rim (arrow). O-P: panoramic and periapical radiograph at six years old showing agenesis of the maxillary lateral incisor on the right.

Case 13

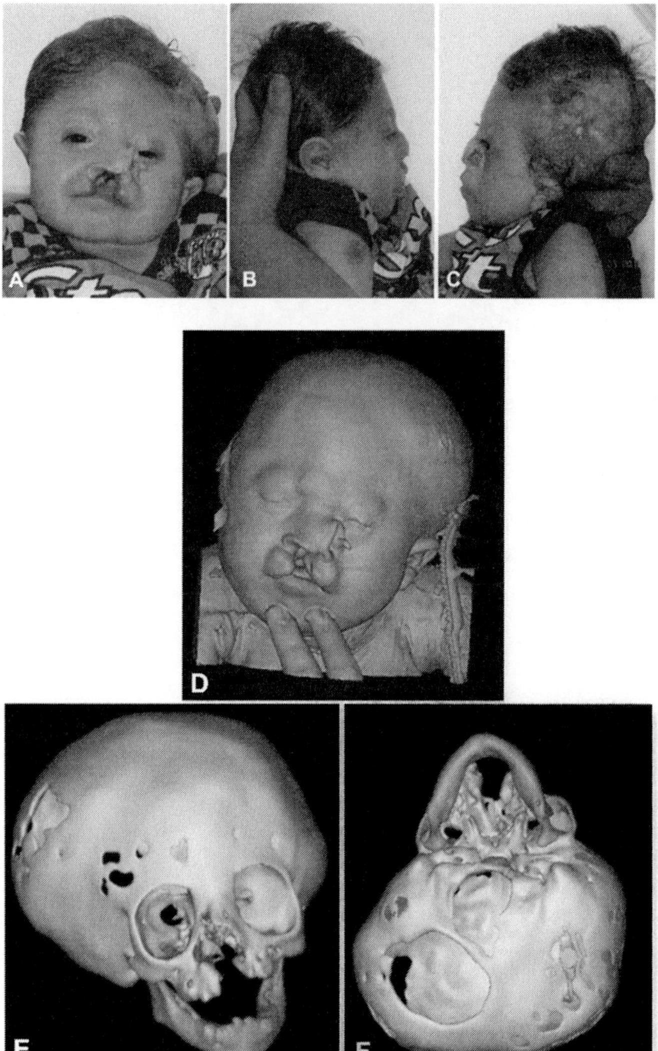

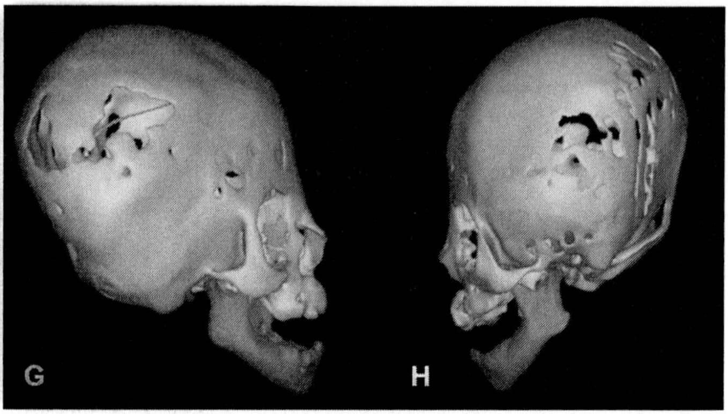

Figure 17– Male patient with a left Tessier cleft number 2 associated with amniotic band sequence. A-C: clinical phenotype at eight months old. Note the turricephaly, prominent metopic suture resembling trigonocephaly, a left wide encephalocele temporoparietal with scalp defect, sparse eyebrows, ocular hypertelorism, ptosis of the right eyelid, facial asymmetry and flat face. The nasal malformation includes asymmetric nasal dorsum, nasal bridge and depressed nasal tip, deviation of the columella to the left, enlarged nostrils, a left alae nasi cleft (Tessier cleft number 2) with a cutaneous appendix inside the nostril and a displacement of the alae nasal to the inner canthus on the left side. Note also a wide right unilateral complete cleft lip and palate. Micrognathia and abnormal ears were observed. D-H: computed tomography was obtained at 12 months old. Figure D is a soft tissue 3D reconstruction showing the facial oro clefts and nasal appendix. Figures E to H are hard tissue 3D reconstructions showing bony failures in the cranium, wide orbital cavities, facial asymmetry, severe midface hypoplasia and short zygomatic arch. A wide right alveolar and palate cleft and a wide right nasal cavity, the nasal septum deviated to the left and Tessier cleft number 2 are observed.

CHAPTER FOUR

TESSIER CLEFT NUMBER 3: THE ORAL-NASAL-OCULAR CLEFT

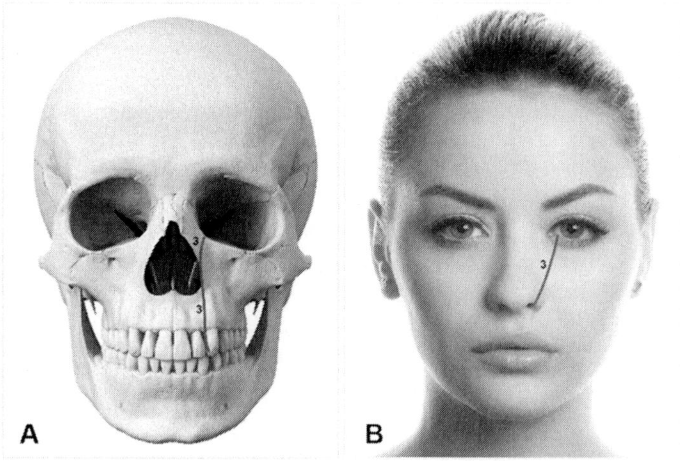

Figure 18 – Localization of Tessier cleft number 3. (A) Bone clefts numbered. (B) Soft tissue clefts numbered. Original artwork by the authors.

Tessier cleft number 3, also called the oral-nasal-ocular cleft, involves the orbit and the lower eyelid in the medial portion. The cleft occurs due to the failure of fusion during the maxillary and lateral nasal processes (Figure 18). Microphthalmia or anophthalmia may occur. The nasal cavity, the nasolacrimal system, the maxillary sinus, the palate and the alveolar arch are affected laterally, resulting in communication between the oral, nasal cavity and the orbit.

References

Allam, K. A., A. A. Lim, A. Elsherbiny, and H. K. Kawamoto. 2014. "The Tessier Number 3 Cleft: A Report of 10 Cases and Review of Literature." *J Plast Reconstr Aesthet Surg* 67 (8): 1055–62. https://doi.org/ 10.1016/j.bjps.2014.04.020.

Da Silva Freitas, R., and Alonso N. Busato. 2010. "Oral-Nasal-Ocular Cleft: The Greatest Challenge among the Rare Clefts." *J Craniofac Surg* 21 (2): 390–95. https://doi.org/ 10.1097/SCS.0b013e3181cfa6b1

David, D. J., M. H. Moore, and R. D. Cooter. 1989. "Tessier Clefts Revisited with a Third Dimension." *Cleft Palate J* 26 (3): 184–85.

Golinko, M. S., J. D. Pemberton, J. Phillips, A. Johnson, and L. D. Hartzell. 2018. "The Arkansas Tessier Number 3 Cleft Experience: Soft Tissue and Skeletal Findings with Primary Surgical Management: Four-Step Approach." *J Craniofac Surg* 29 (7): 1834–41. https://doi.org/ 10.1097/SCS.0000000000004634

Morgan, A. L., R. Cason, and El Amm. 2016. "Anthropometrically Based Surgical Technique for Tessier 3 Cleft Reconstruction." *J Craniofac Surg* 27 (8): e785–87. https://doi.org/10.1097/SCS.0000000000003129.

Tessier, Paul. 1976. "Anatomical Classification of Facial, Cranio-Facial and Latero-Facial Clefts." *Journal of Maxillofacial Surgery* 4: 69–92. https://doi.org/10.1016/s0301-0503(76)80013-6.

Tessier cleft number 3

Case 14

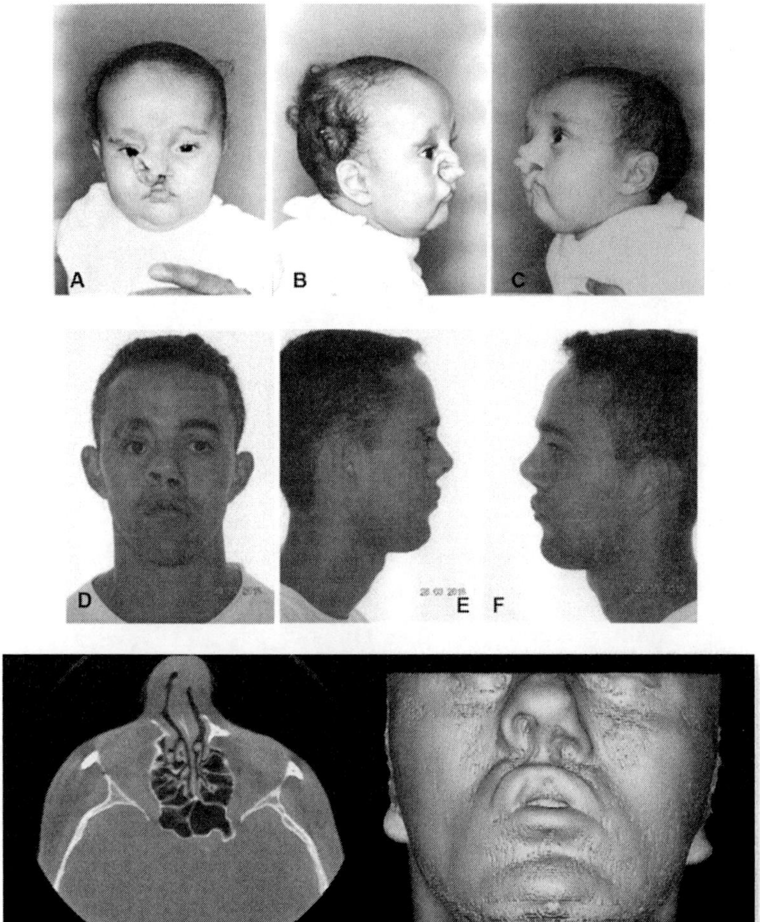

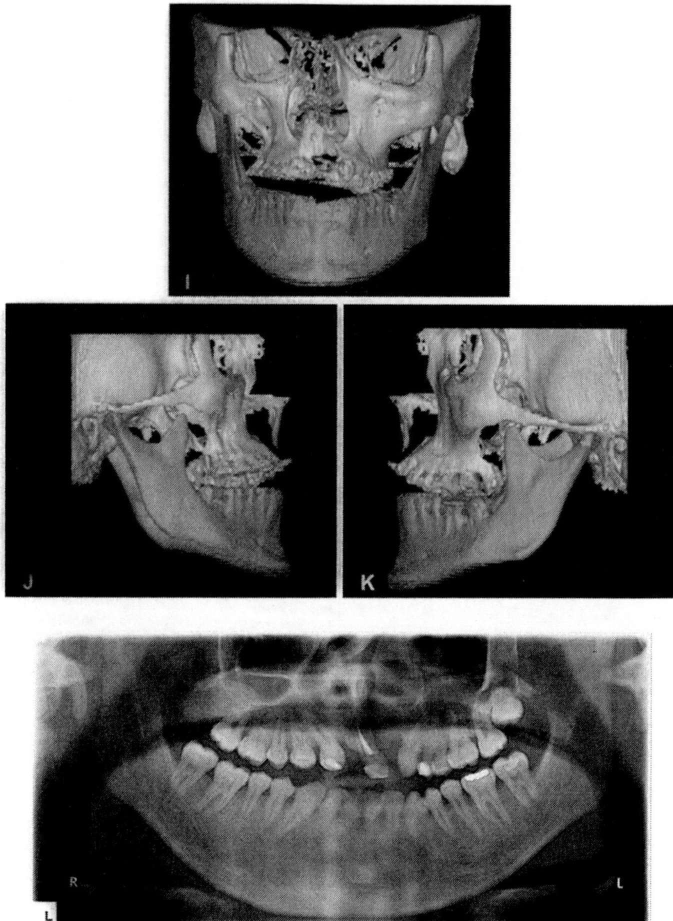
I
J
K
R
L
L

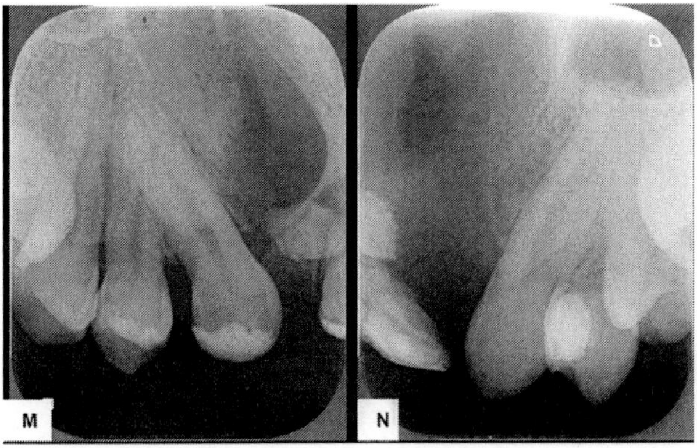

Figure 19 – Clinical phenotype of a male patient with a Tessier cleft number 3 on the right side. A-C: At eight months old, observe a wide forehead, a notch in the right eyebrow, and a bilateral complete cleft lip on the left and palate. The right cleft lip extended into the nasal cavity, dragging the nasal alae to the inner canthus lacrimal punctum (Tessier cleft number 3). The nose has deviated to the right with a narrow nasal tip. D-F: facial phenotype at age 21 showing a mild facial asymmetry with a right smaller eye and a notch of the upper lid and eyebrow (Tessier cleft number 11). The orofacial cleft was repaired, demonstrating a short philtrum, columella and a prominent premaxilla with an everted upper lip. F: computed tomography axial section showing deviation of the nasal tip and septum. H-K: computed tomography 3D reconstructions obtained at 22 years old. Observe the bone tissue showing a wide nasal cavity with a protruded premaxilla and notch in the frontal process of the maxilla (arrow). L-N: panoramic and periapical radiograph at 20 years old showing agenesis of teeth 12, 21 and 22 in periapical image note bilateral maxillary alveolar defect.

Case 15

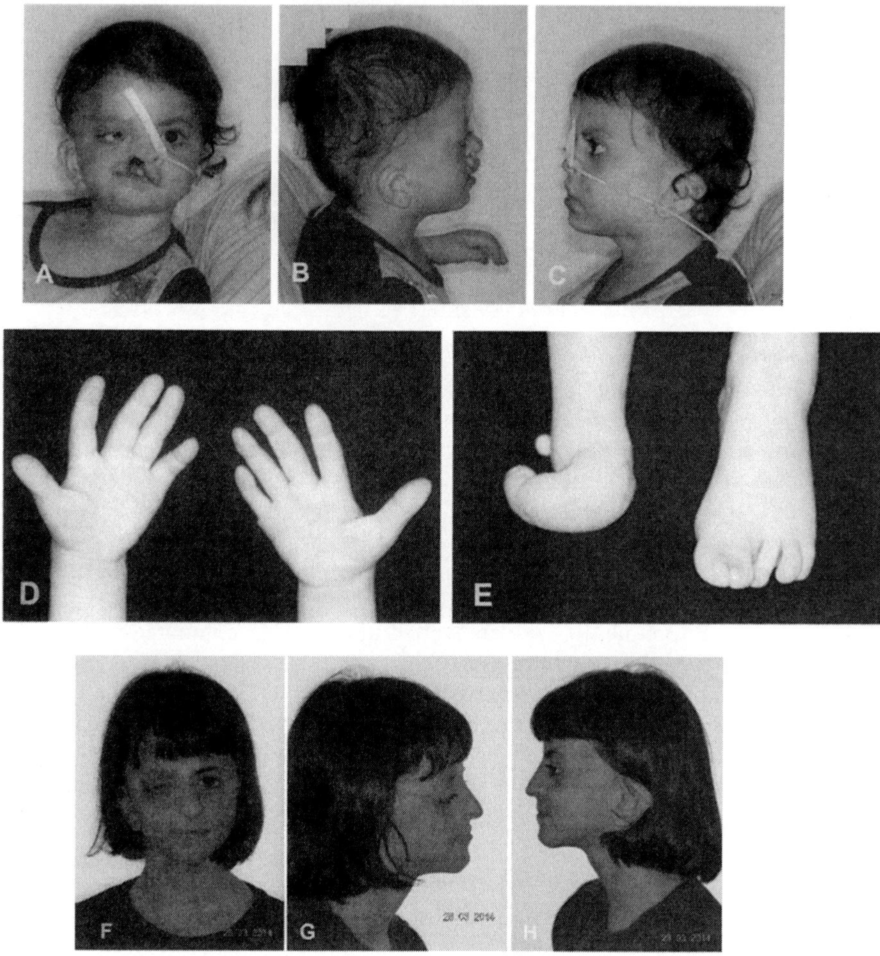

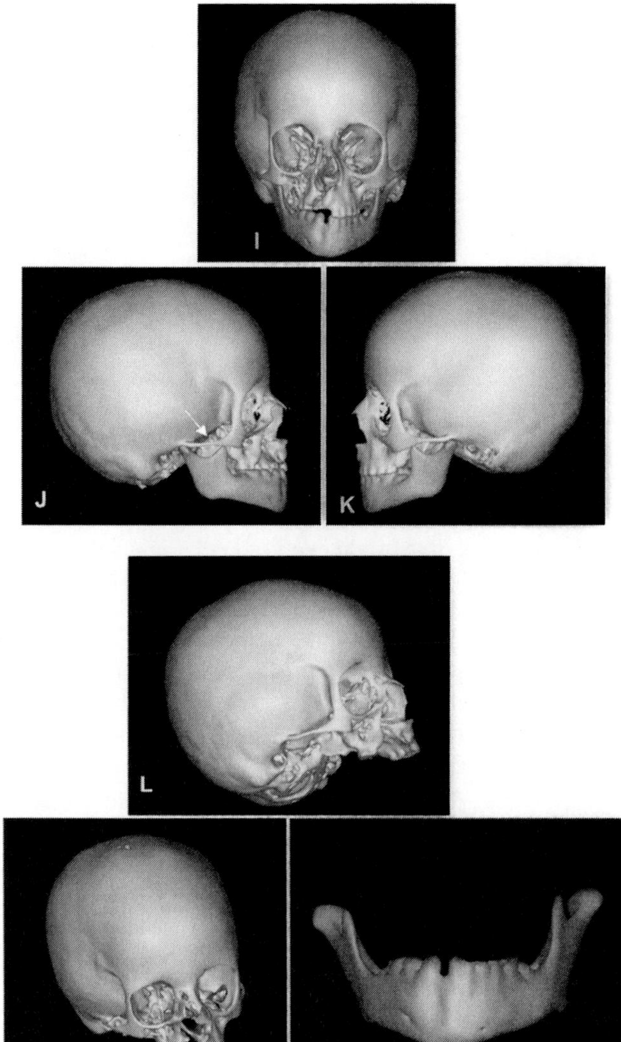
I
J
K
L
M
N

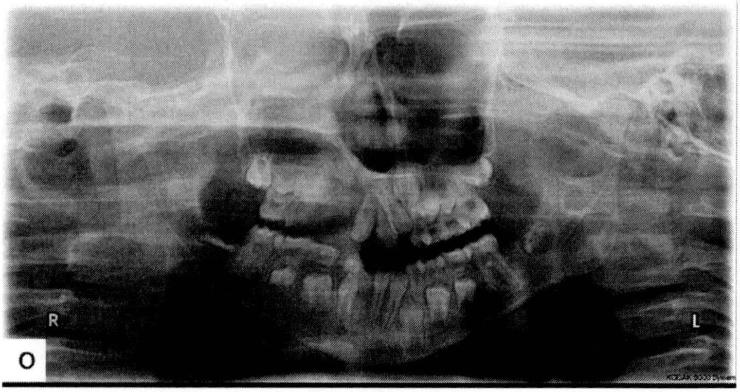

Figure 20 – Clinical phenotype of a female patient with Goltz-Gorlin syndrome (OMIM 305600) and Tessier cleft number 3. A-C: at six months old, note the wide forehead, right complete cleft lip and palate associated with an oral-nasal-ocular cleft (Tessier number 3), an ocular anomaly (microphthalmia, ptosis of the right eyelid) on the right side, and prominent and low-set ears. D-E: hand and feet photographs. Note bilateral thumb low implantation and ungueal dysplasia of the fingers, duplication of the hallux on the left side, and oligodactyly on the right foot. F-H: facial phenotype at age nine. Note the sparse eyebrow on the right side, ocular abnormality on the right, ocular hypertelorism, mild facial asymmetry, narrow nasal bridge, wide nasal tip, and a notched nasal ala. I-N: computed tomography 3D reconstructions obtained at nine years old showing a right oral cleft extending to the wide nasal cavity and orbital region with a hypoplastic nasal bone on the right side (Tessier cleft number 3), a hypoplastic zygomatic arch (arrow), and a mandibular cleft (Tessier cleft number 30). Figure L is a lateral view of the right side showing the hypoplasia of the medial orbital rim and hypoplasia of the zygomatic bone and maxilla. Figure M demonstrates the alveolar cleft, cleft palate and the communication between the orbit, maxillary sinus and nose. Figure N reveals more details of the median mandibular cleft (Tessier cleft number 30). O: Panoramic radiograph at age eight shows agenesis of the maxillary lateral incisor and canine (12–13) on the right and agenesis of the mandibular central and lateral incisors (41–42) on the right.

Case 16

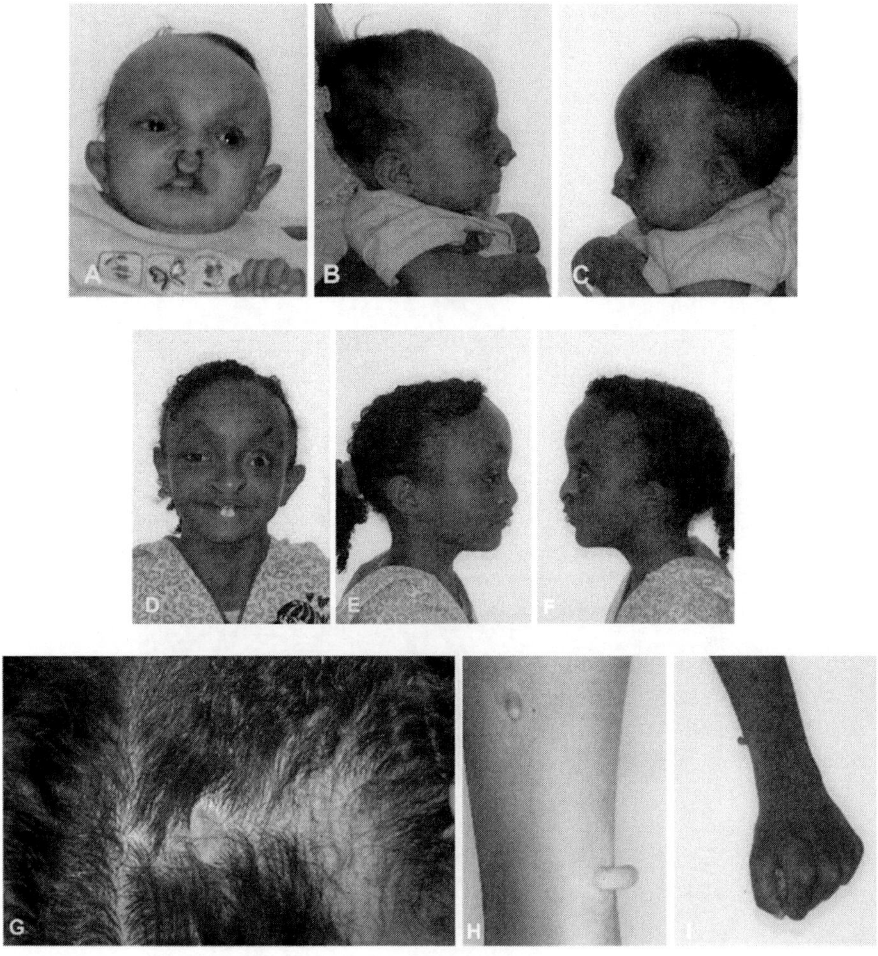

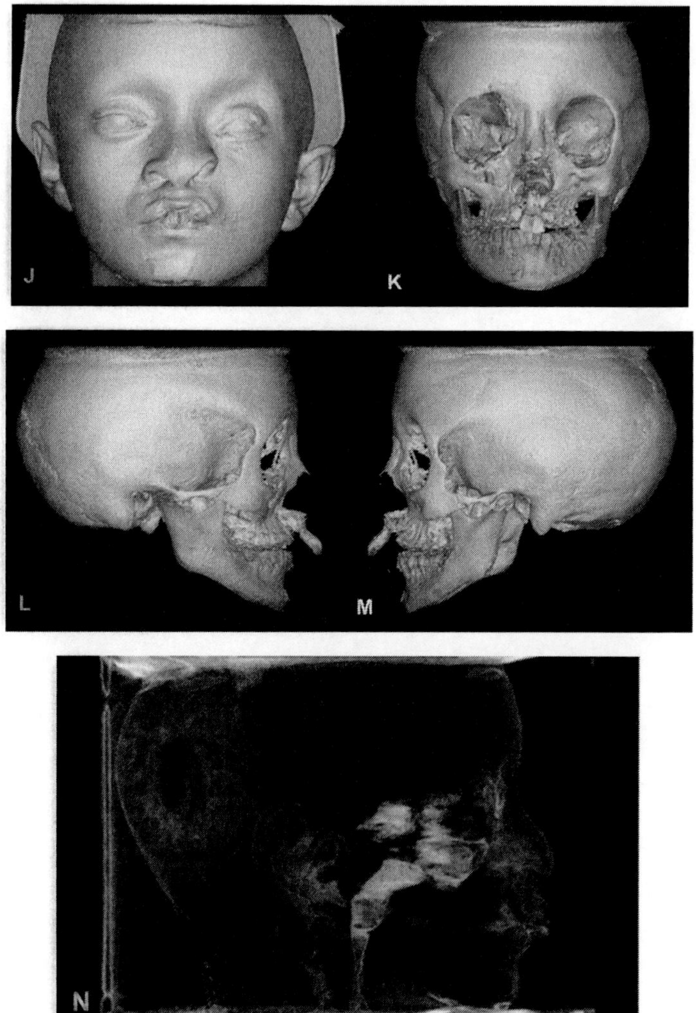

Figure 21 – Clinical phenotype of a female patient with Amniotic Band sequence/Disorganization and Tessier cleft number 3. A-C: At four months old, note the broad forehead, the ocular hypertelorism, the arched and sparse eyebrows, a coloboma of the medial portion of the upper eyelid on the left side (Tessier cleft number 11), a bilateral complete cleft lip and palate extending to the nasal and ocular regions (Tessier cleft number 3) on the left and a protruded and low-set ears. D-F: facial phenotype at ten years old.

Observe the wide forehead with no hair in the anterior midline and parietal area (frontal balding), an abnormal medial portion of the eyebrow bilaterally, mostly marked on the left side. A left upper palpebral coloboma was observed, extending as a notch to the medial portion of the eyebrow and parietal region (Tessier cleft number 11). An asymmetric and flat nose, a short columella, a prominent premaxilla, an interposition of maxillary central incisors between the upper and lower lips and abnormal ears were present. G: failure of scalp hair. H-I: left arm. Note the congenital skin pedicles. J-M: computed tomography 3D images obtained at ten years old. In Figure J, at the level of the soft tissue, note the notch in the supraorbital region, palpebral coloboma and alae nasi hypoplasia in a continuous line with the repaired oral cleft on the left (arrow - Tessier cleft numbers 3 and 11) and the repaired oral cleft on the right side. In figures K to M, observe the broad orbital cavity, the absence of bony clefting of the supraorbital rim, the midface hypoplasia and the short and hypoplastic zygomatic arch. N: the upper airway space in the lateral view demonstrated a narrow oropharynx.

Case 17

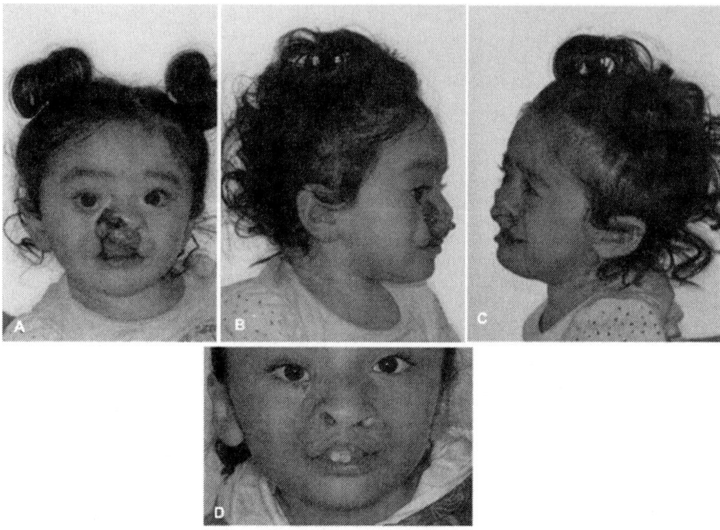

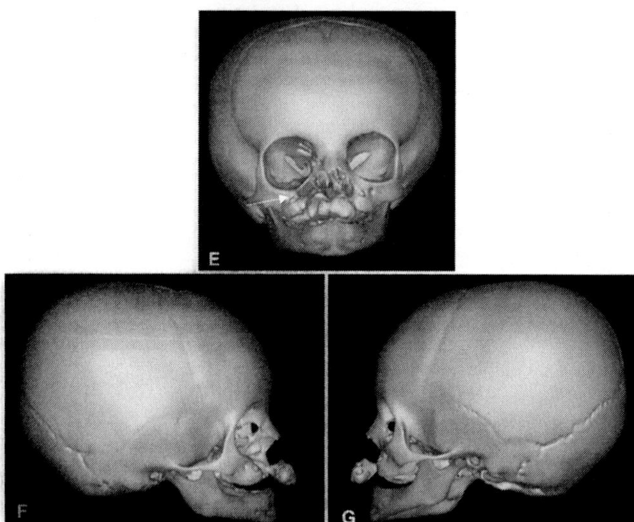

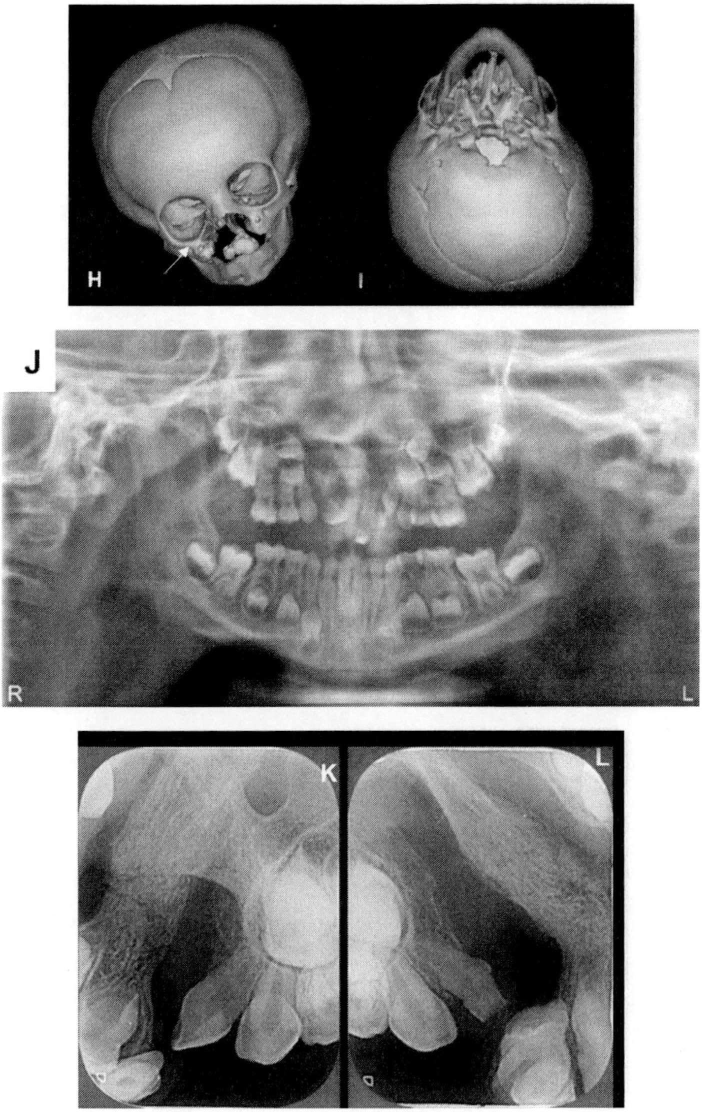

Figure 22 – Female patient with a Tessier cleft number 3 with amniotic band sequence. A-E: clinical phenotype at ten months old. Note in the soft tissue a left cleft lip and palate, a wide right oral cleft with absent septation between the nasal cavity and maxillary affecting the nose until the medial canthus of the lower lid (Tessier cleft number 3). D: facial photographs at

three years old showing the repaired clefts. E-I: computed tomography obtained at 12 months showing the protruded premaxilla, a wide nasal cavity and communication between the oral cavity, the nasal cavity, and the infraorbital rim representing the right oro-naso-ocular cleft (arrow - Tessier number 3). A left alveolar cleft is also observed.

J: panoramic radiograph at seven years old showing agenesis of the bilateral maxillary lateral incisors (12–22). K-L: periapical radiograph at seven years old shows an alveolar defect in the maxillary arch.

Case 18

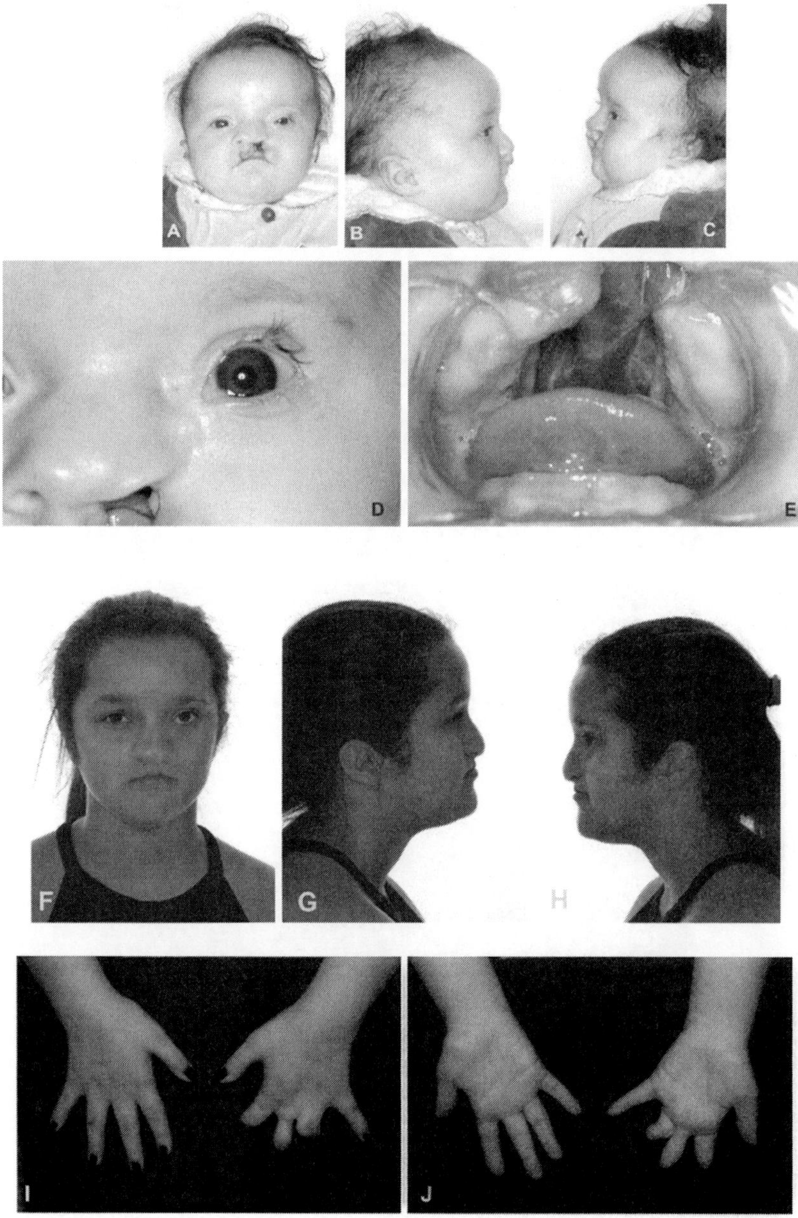

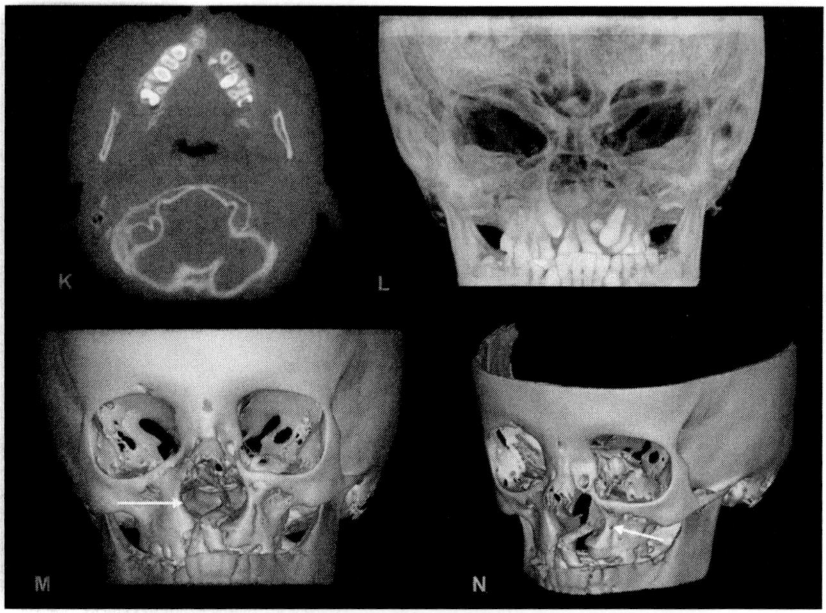
K
L
M
N

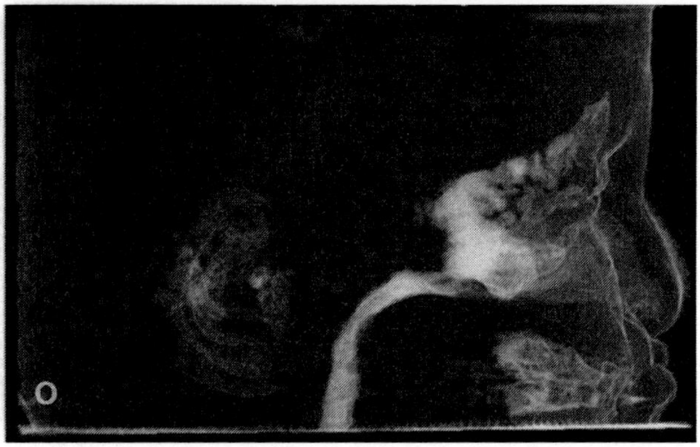
O

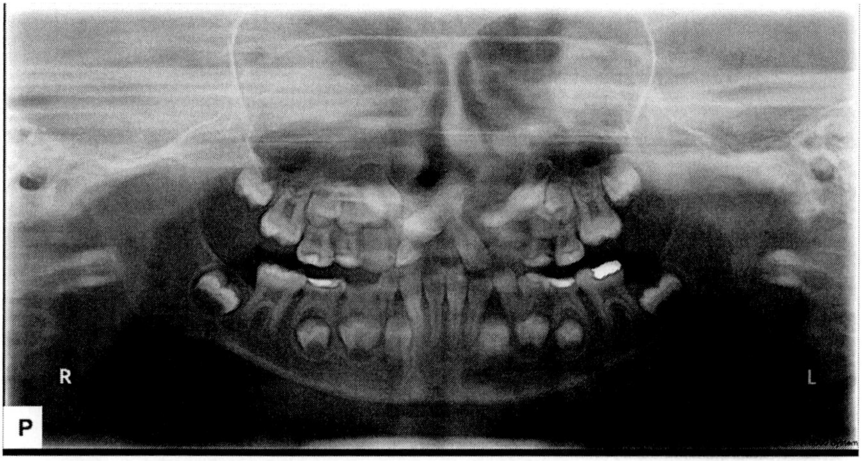

Figure 23 – Clinical phenotype of a female patient with amniotic band sequence and Tessier cleft number 3. A-E: at eight months old, note the broad forehead, the ocular hypertelorism and a short and abnormal palpebral fissure with coloboma in the left upper eyelid. Observe the right cleft lip, a complete left cleft lip and palate extending to the alae nasi until the inner canthus of the lower eyelid, and the medial to inferior lacrimal punctum (Tessier cleft number 3). In Figure D, note the cleft of the medial region of the upper eyelid and the irregularity in eyelash orientation and in Figure E, the cleft in an alveolar ridge on the left and cleft palate. F-H: facial phenotype at 11 years old. Note the mild face asymmetry on the left side with a cicatricial notch extending to the oral and ocular regions. The nose is flattened with a wide and depressed nasal tip, and the columella and philtrum are shortened. I-J: hands of the patient. Note the hypoplasia of the second–fourth fingers on the left hand with a mild ring constriction on the third digit. K-L: computed tomography-derived images obtained at eight years old. Figure K is an axial section showing the left alveolar cleft. Figure L illustrates a translucent 3D reconstruction showing the asymmetric maxilla. Figures M to N show a wide nasal bridge, a nasal septum deviation, an oral cleft extending to the maxillary sinus, nasal cavity, and lower orbital rim (Tessier cleft number 3 in the bone structure). A midface hypoplasia, a prominent premaxilla and a Class III skeletal and dental relationship are present; the upper incisors are vertical with an anterior crossbite. O: the upper airway lateral view reveals a narrow naso and oropharynx. P: panoramic radiograph at six years old showing agenesis of bilateral maxillary lateral incisors (12 and 22), supernumerary teeth adjacent to cleft regions (13 and 23) and alveolar defects (between 11–13 and 21–23).

CHAPTER FIVE

TESSIER CLEFT NUMBER 4: THE OCULO-FACIAL-CLEFT (CENTRAL ORBITO-MAXILLARY CLEFT)

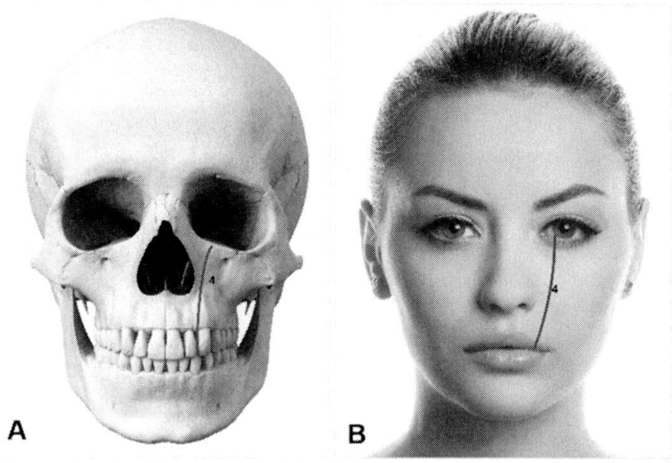

Figure 24 – Localization of Tessier cleft number 4. (A) Bone clefts numbered. (B) Soft tissue clefts numbered. Original artwork by the authors.

Tessier cleft number 4, or oculofacial cleft, involves the upper lip and philtrum, the medial region of the maxillary sinus to the lower margin of the orbit, and there is no involvement of the nose and the nasolacrimal system (Figure 24). In cases where the alveolar region is affected, the cleft passes between the lateral incisors and the canines. The soft tissue of the middle third of the face is quite deficient. In addition, the alae nasi is displaced to the upper part of the face and the nose is shortened.

References

Alonso N, Freitas R da S, de Oliveira e Cruz GA, Goldenberg D, Dall'oglioTolazzi AR. Tessier nº. 4 facial cleft: evolution of surgical treatment in a large series of patients. *Plast Reconstr Surg*. 2008;122(5):1505-1513. https://doi.org/ 10.1097/PRS.0b013e318188209c.

Caruso, P. A., G. J. Harris, and B. L. Padwa. 2003. "CT Imaging of Craniofacial Malformations." *Neuroimaging Clin N Am* 13 (3): 541–72. https://doi.org/10.1016/s1052-5149(03)00061-3.

Cannistrà, Claudio, Claire Bontemps, Rodrigo Valero, Giorgio Iannetti and J. Patrick Barbet. 2006. "Orbitofacial Cleft Number 5: Radiographic, Anatomical and Histologic Study of a 24-Week-Old Fetus." *Plastic and Reconstructive Surgery* 118 (7): 1538–42. https://doi.org/10.1097/01.prs.0000240818.64018.2a.

David, D. J., M. H. Moore, and R. D. Cooter. 1989. "Tessier Clefts Revisited with a Third Dimension." *Cleft Palate J* 26 (3): 184–85.

Rahpeyma, A., and S. Khajehahmadi. 2015. "Treatment of a Unilateral Tessier Number 4 Facial Cleft in an Adult: Role of Nasolabial V-Y Advancement Flap." *Br J Oral Maxillofac Surg* 53 (1): 99–101. https://doi.org/ 10.1016/j.bjoms.2014.09.019.

Tessier, Paul. 1976. "Anatomical Classification of Facial, Cranio-Facial and Latero-Facial Clefts." *Journal of Maxillofacial Surgery* 4: 69–92. https://doi.org/10.1016/s0301-0503(76)80013-6.

Winters, Ryan. 2016. "Tessier Clefts and Hypertelorism". *Facial Plastic Surgery Clinics of North America* 24 (4): 545–58. https://doi.org/10.1016/j.fsc.2016.06.013.

Tessier cleft number 4

Case 19

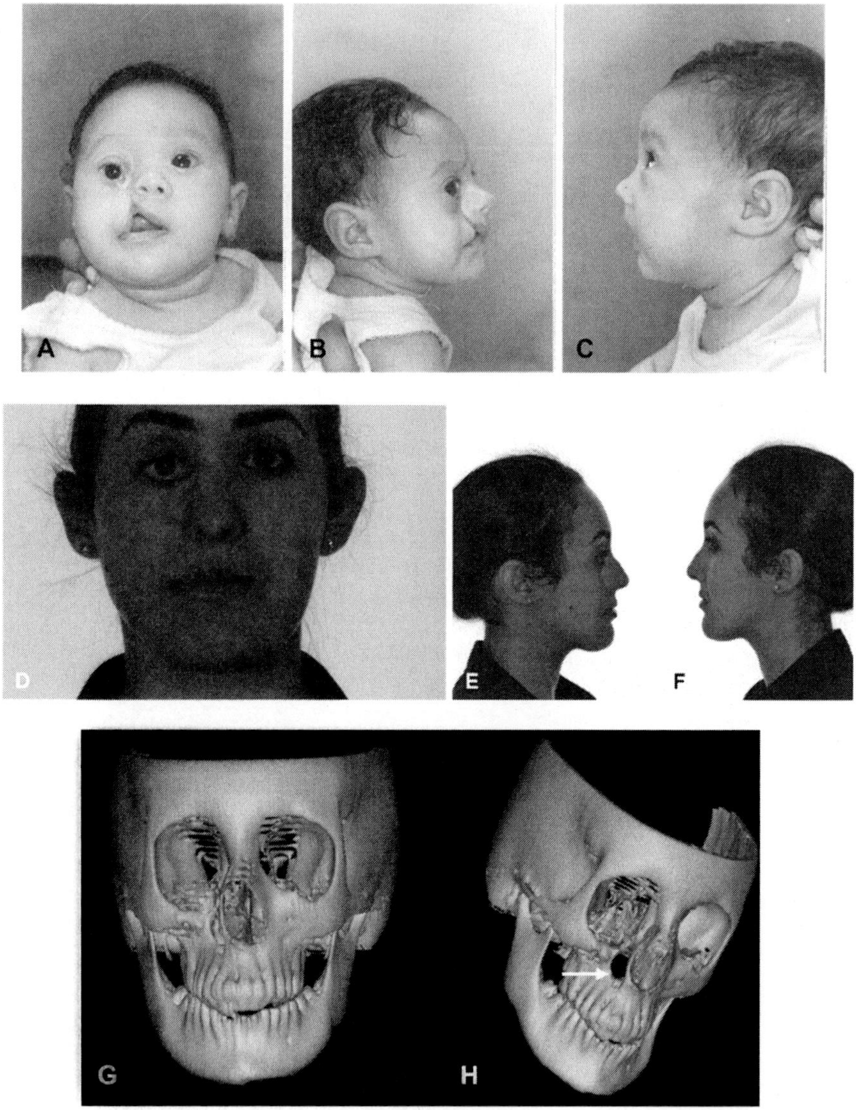

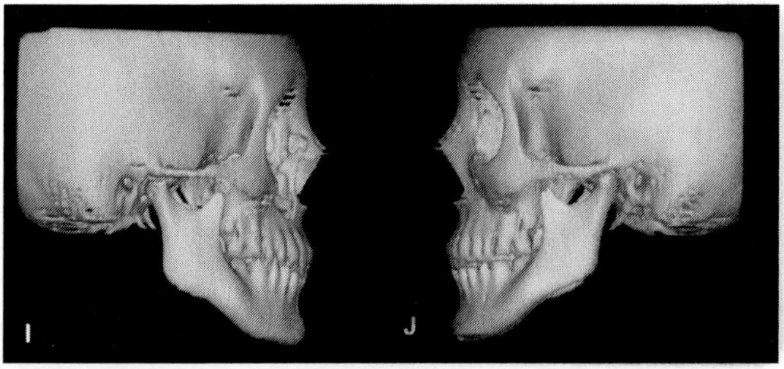

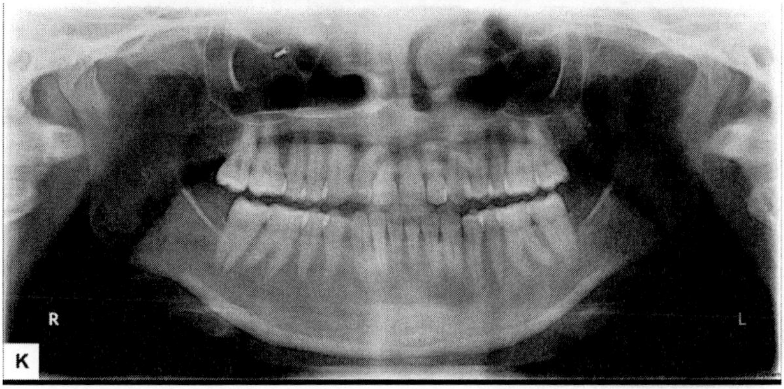

Figure 25 – Clinical phenotype of a female patient with a classic Tessier cleft number 4. A-C: At 11 months old, note the right cleft lip and oculofacial cleft (Tessier number 4). The nasal alae are anatomically normal and superiorly displaced. D-F: facial phenotype at 25 years old showing the repaired cleft and an ocular asymmetry. G-J: computed tomography 3D reconstructions obtained at age 18 showed a midface hypoplasia on the right side. A cleft around the pyriform aperture through the medial maxillary sinus was observed until the infraorbital foramen and lower orbital rim (arrow). K: panoramic radiograph at 24 years old showing no dental anomalies and alveolar defects between 12–13.

Case 20

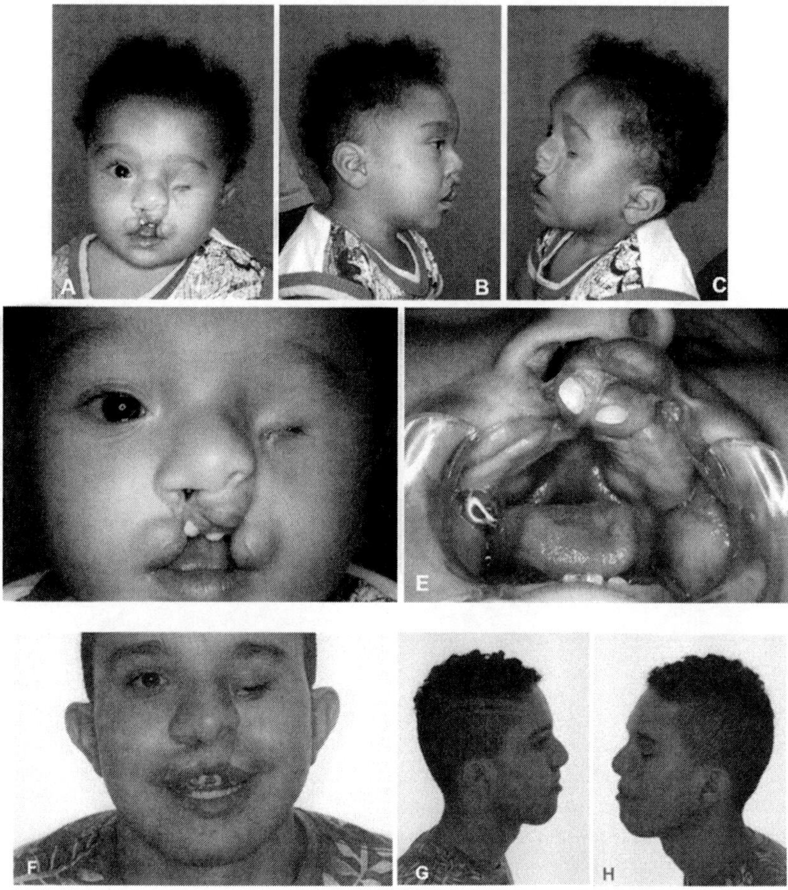

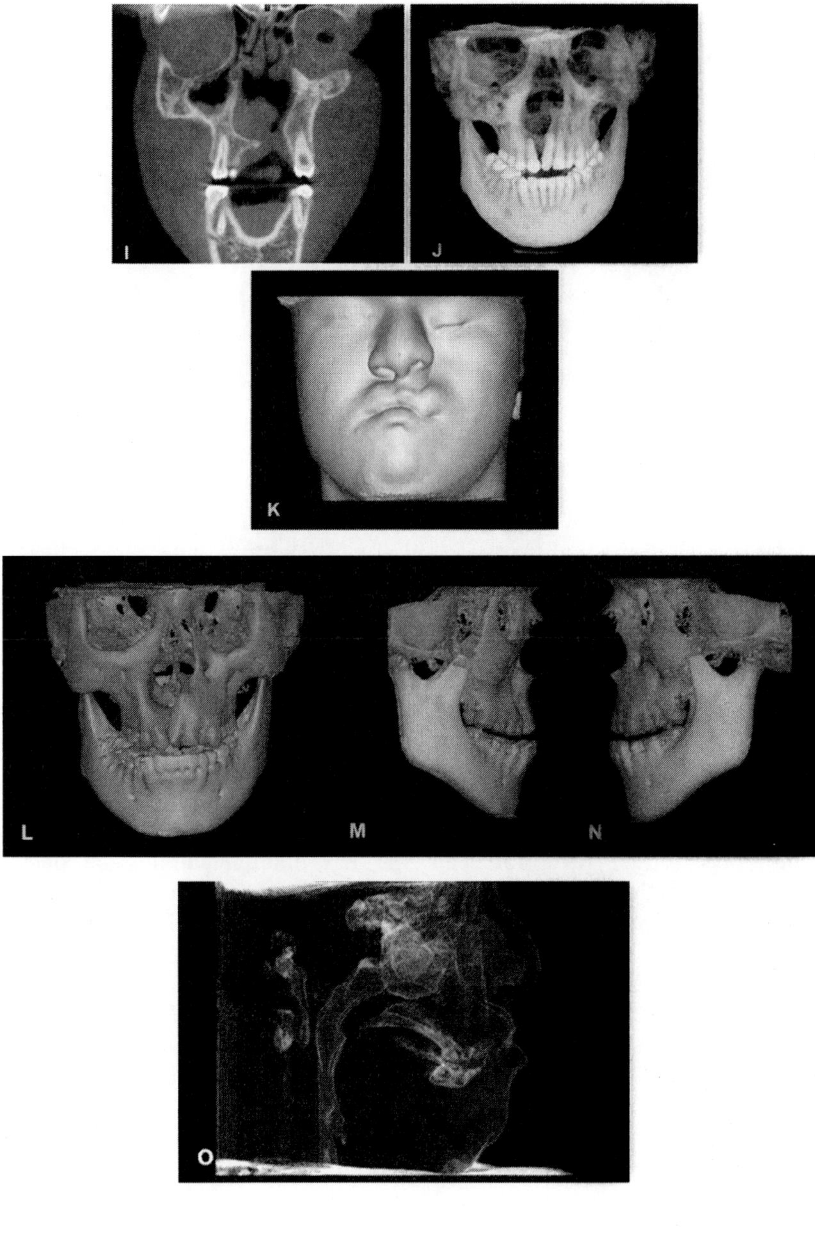
I
J
K
L
M
N
O

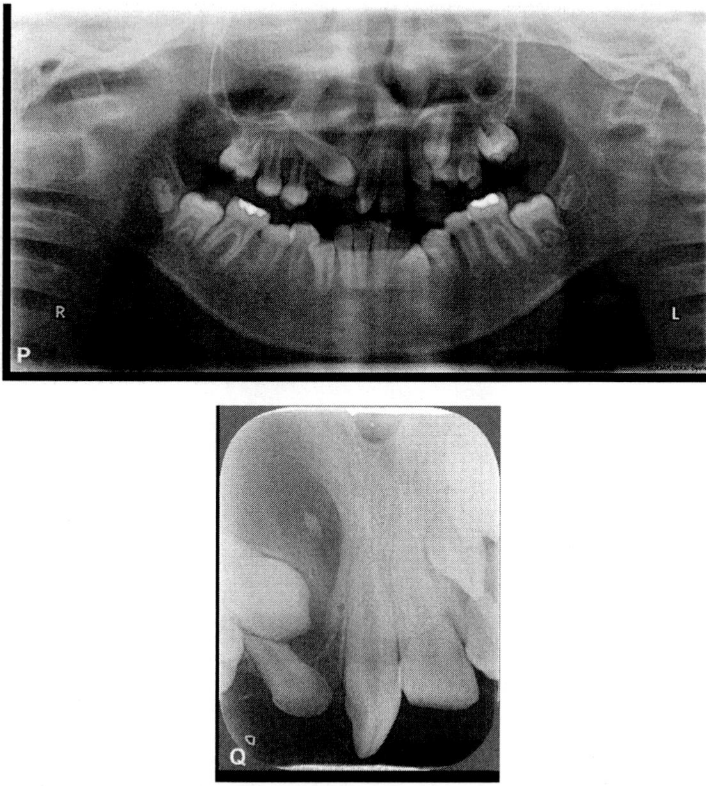

Figure 26 – Male patient with Tessier cleft number 4. A-E: at 11 months old, observe the wide forehead, the left microphthalmia, the ocular hypertelorism, the depressed nasal bridge, the nasal tip with deviation to the left, the short columella, the right cleft lip and alveolus, and the left cleft lip extending to the medial canthus of the eye as a notch (Tessier cleft number 4). Observe that the nasal alae are not involved. Figure D shows the cleft lip and the oral-ocular cleft with microphthalmia and ankyloblepharon, and Figure E shows a cleft in the alveolar arch on the right and a notch on the left. E-G: facial phenotype at age 16. Observe the left short palpebral fissure with ptosis, a repaired ankyloblepharon and a repaired cleft lip and oro-ocular cleft. H-M: computed tomography images obtained at 15 years old. Figure H is a coronal section showing a reduced left orbital cavity and nasal septum deviation. Figure I is a translucent 3D reconstruction demonstrating a short nasal cavity length with an incomplete cleft lip and micro dent on the left side, a right alveolar cleft with a large nasal cavity and agenesis of

the right maxillary lateral incisor. Figure J demonstrates the nasal asymmetry remaining after surgical repairs. Figures K to N reveal a decreased length of the left orbital cavity, a hypoplastic maxillary bone in the infraorbital rim region and a larger left maxillary sinus. A mild alveolar notch extending to the maxillary sinus on the left and an alveolar cleft on the right is also observed. O: the upper airway lateral view demonstrated a normal image. P: panoramic radiograph at ten years old showing agenesis of the maxillary lateral incisors (12) and (O) a periapical radiograph showing the maxillary alveolar defect between the central incisor and canine (11-13) on the right.

Case 21

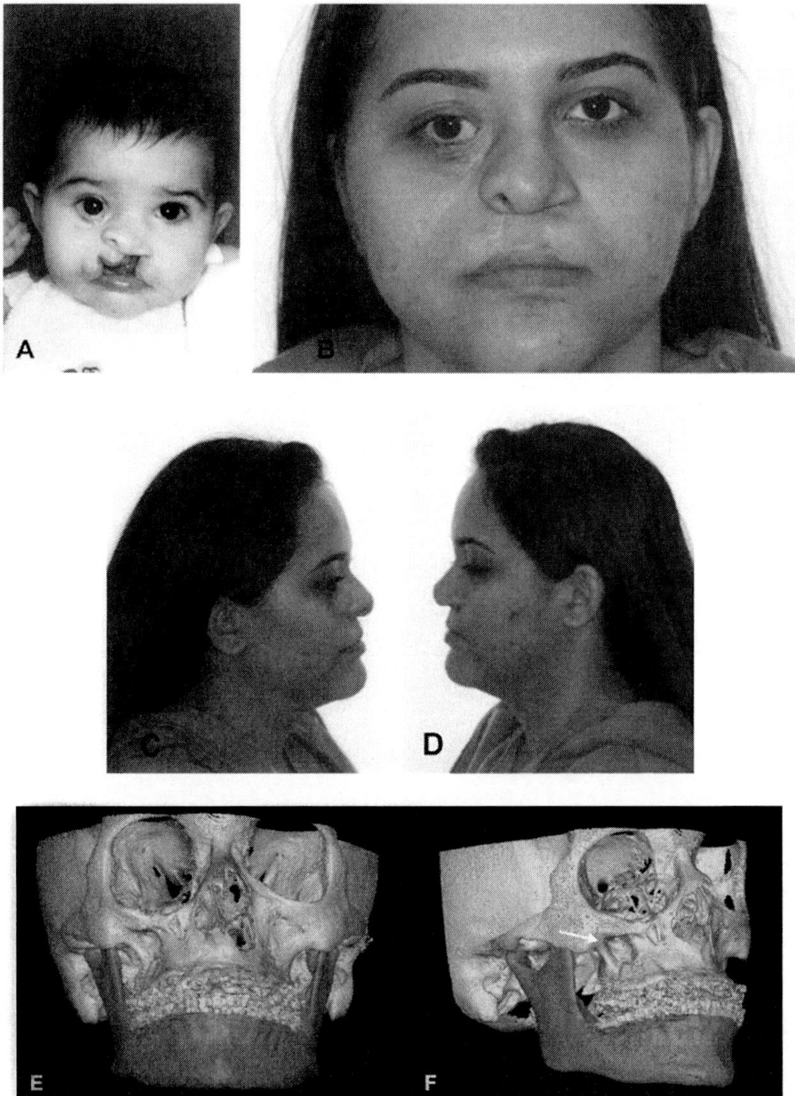

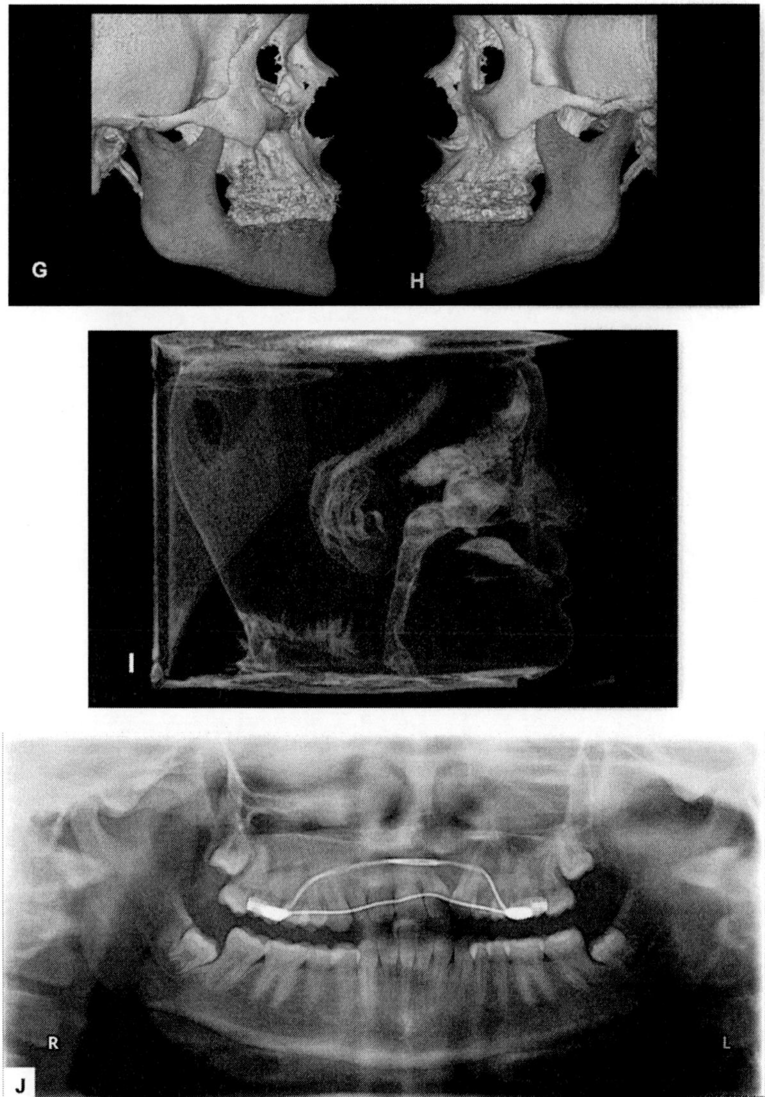

Figure 27–Female patient with a Tessier cleft number 4. A: clinical phenotype at six months old. Note in the soft tissue a right incomplete cleft lip extending to the ocular region as a notch, ending in a palpebral coloboma in the lower eyelid lateral to the punctum (Tessier cleft number 4). A complete left cleft lip was present, with a depressed nasal tip associated with

a columella deviated to the right. The records registered an incomplete cleft in the soft palate (clinical find not shown in the picture). B-D: facial photographs at 23 years old showing the repaired cleft, a slight asymmetry orbit, midface hypoplasia on the right side and asymmetrical nasal alae. E-H: computed tomography 3D reconstructions obtained at age 21 showing lower orbital rim hypoplasia, a zygomatic bone (arrow) failure, and asymmetry in the nasal cavity. I: the upper airway lateral view demonstrated a normal image. J: panoramic radiograph at 17 years old showing agenesis of the maxillary lateral incisor (22), supernumerary teeth between 12–13 and bilateral alveolar defects (12–13 and 21–23).

Case 22

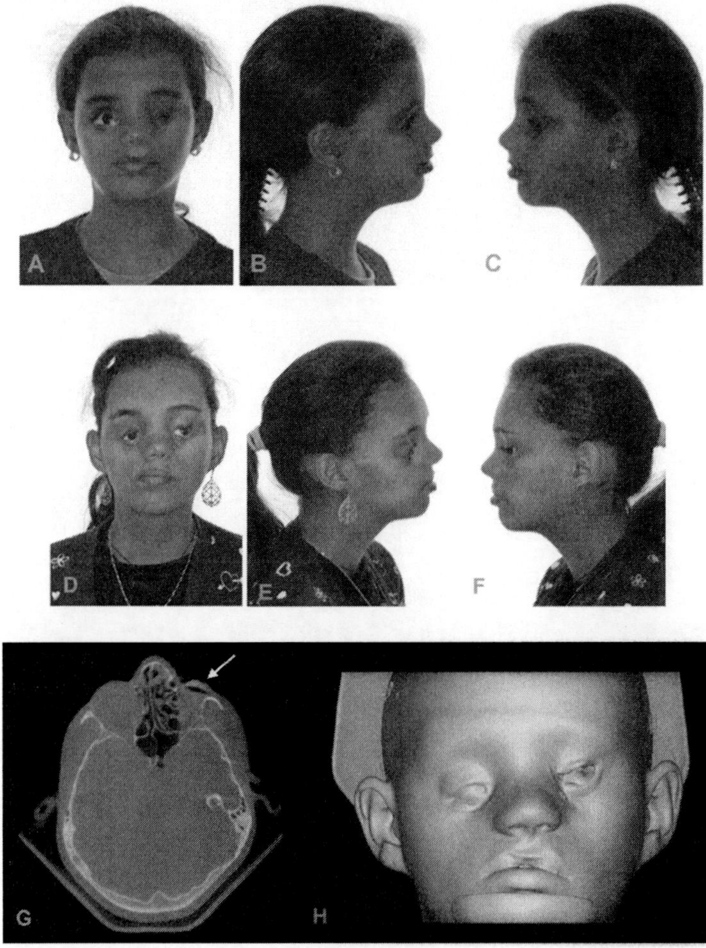

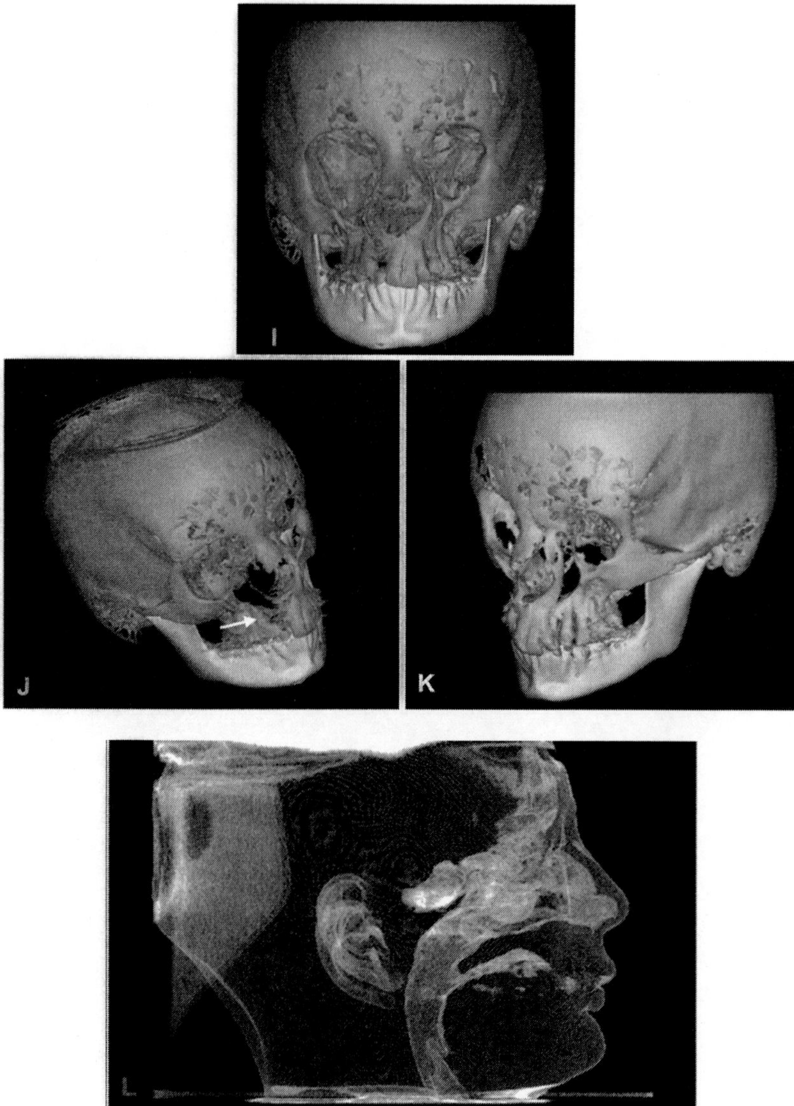
I
J
K
L

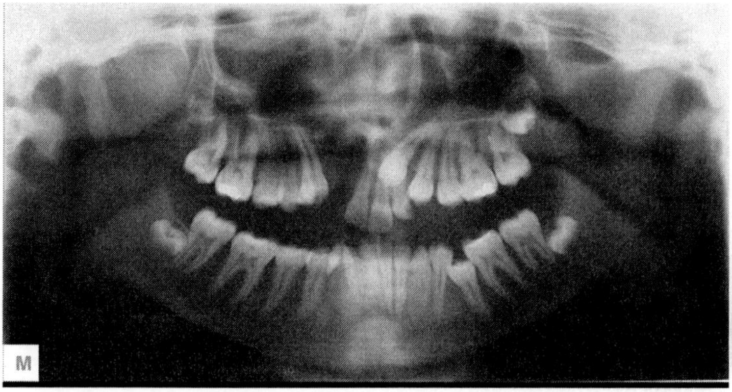

Figure 28– Female patient demonstrating a bilateral Tessier cleft number 4. A-C: clinical phenotype at ten years old. Note the microphthalmia (on the left side with an irregular border of the palpebral fissure and abnormal implantation of eyelashes like colobomas). A surgical scar was present in the outer corner of the eyelid. On the right side, observe a lower palpebral irregularly with a tissue-like cornea (epibulbar dermoid) in the inner canthus and the absence of the outer canthus (Tessier cleft number eight). A surgical scar extended to the temporal region. A short nose with hypoplasia of the nostrils was present. Note a complete bilateral cleft lip and palate associated with a cleft lip extending to the ocular region as a notch finishing in a lower palpebral irregularity laterally to the lacrimal punctum (Tessier cleft number 4). D-F: facial phenotype at 16 years old showing a midface and ocular facial asymmetry. Note the presence of an ocular prosthesis on the left side. G-L: computed tomography was obtained at 27 years old. Figure G is an axial section showing the nasal septum deviation and microphthalmia (arrow). In Figure H, the soft tissue reconstruction shows a short philtrum. Three-dimensional reconstructions of the skeletal tissue in figures I to K demonstrate a failure in the frontal bone (copper-beaten skull) and a short left orbital cavity. A wide cleft starting at the alveolar region (arrow) between the lateral incisor and canine on both sides extends to the medial region of the maxillary sinus until the infraorbital foramen and the lower orbital rim around the pyriform aperture. L: the upper airway space in the lateral view had a normal and wide morphology. M: panoramic radiograph at 11 years old showing agenesis of the maxillary lateral incisor (12) and bilateral alveolar defects (11–13 and 22–23).

Case 23

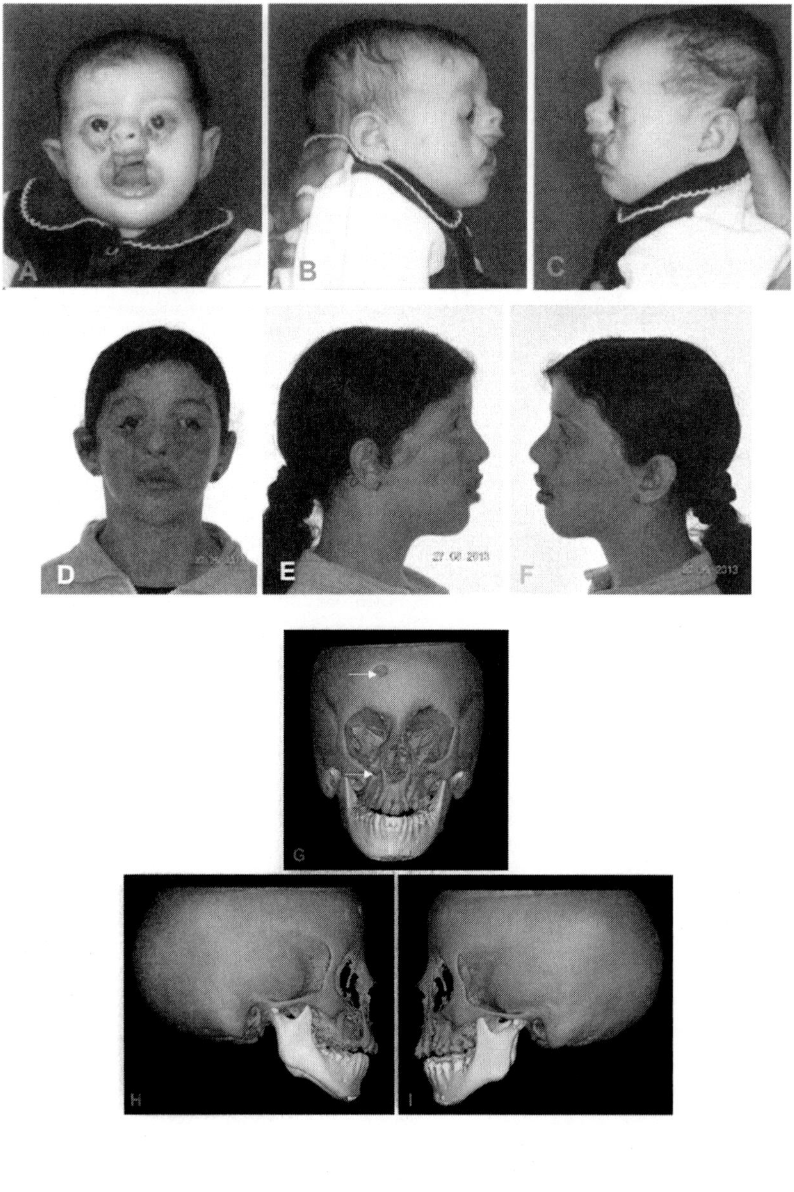

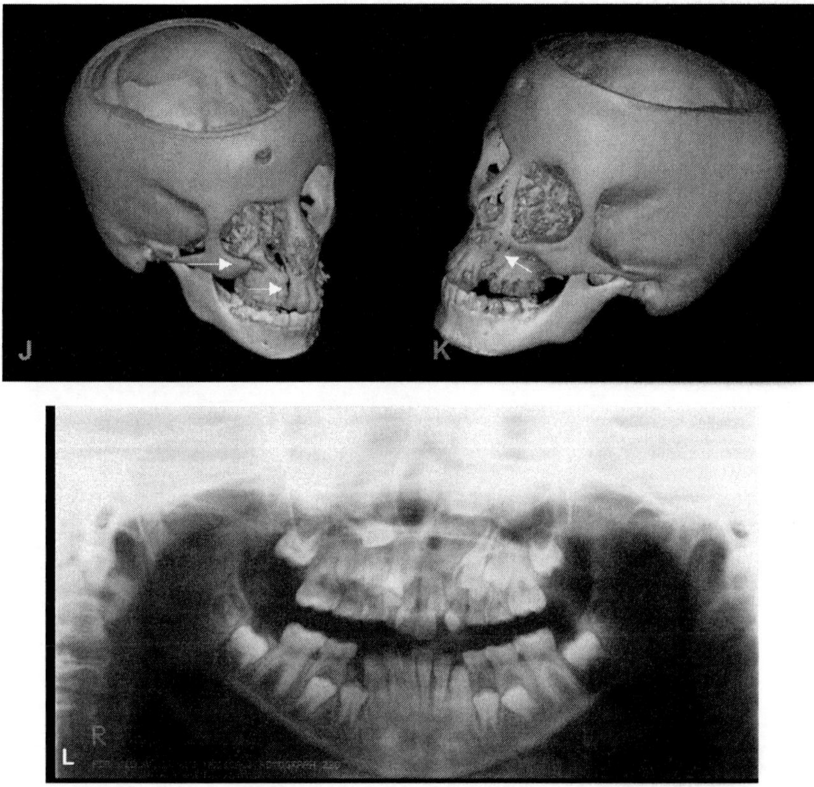

Figure 29– Female patient with a bilateral Tessier cleft number 4. A-C: clinical phenotype at five months old. Note the presence of a broad forehead with small frontal cele (meningoencephalocele) on the right side, sparse eyebrows and down-slanted palpebral fissures. An abnormal upper eyelid (inner canthus in the medial region of the eyelid) with an absence of eyelashes bilaterally, wide lower lid ectropion with wide coloboma bilaterally dragging the infraorbital rim down and decreasing the oro-ocular distance was observed. A short nose length and a cleft lip and palate extending to the inner palpebral coloboma as a notch bilaterally (Tessier cleft number 4) were seen. A lateral cleft (Tessier cleft number 7) is present bilaterally. D-F: facial phenotype at 13 years old showing repaired clefts and midface hypoplasia. G-K: computed tomography 3D reconstructions obtained at age 12. Observe the bitemporal narrowing, a bone failure in the frontal bone on the right side (arrow), a wide orbital cavity and a deviation of the nasal bone to the right side. An alveolar cleft between the lateral

incisor and canine extending to the orbital region (Tessier cleft number 4) is present on both sides. In the oblique view (Figures J and K), observe a wide Tessier cleft number 4 on the right side with an alveolar cleft and a wide orbital floor cleft (arrow). On the left side, the alveolar cleft passes through the frontal process of the maxilla until the lower orbital rim, which is hypoplastic. L: panoramic radiograph at eight years old showing an absence of dental anomalies

Case 24

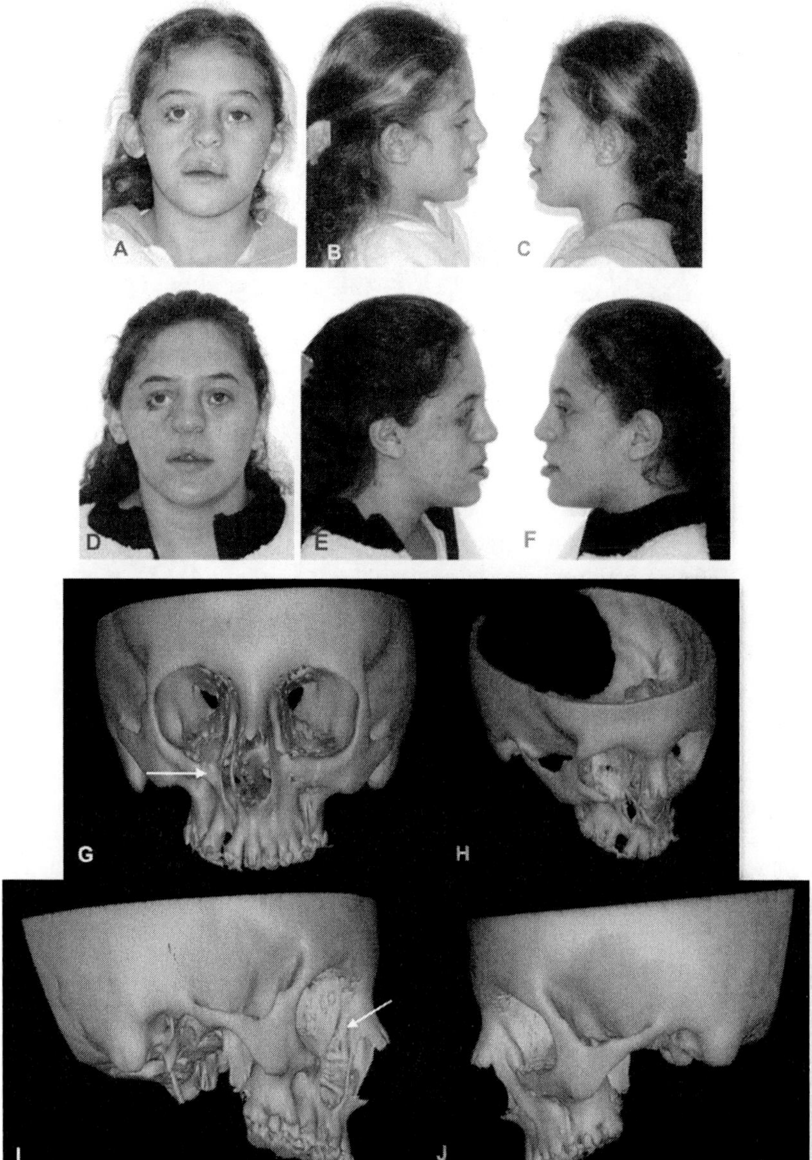

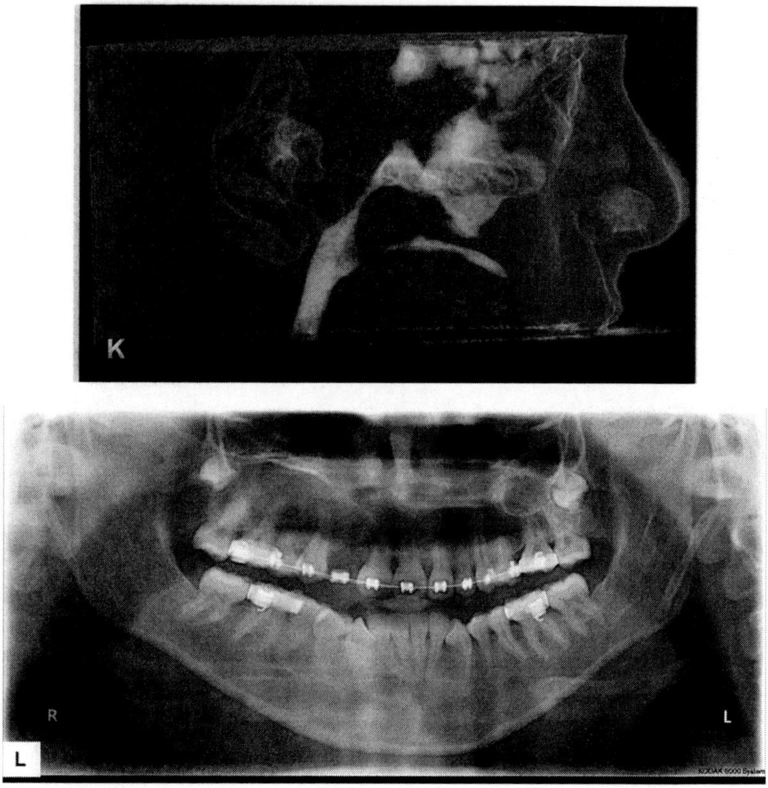

Figure 30 – Female patient with a bilateral Tessier cleft number 4. A-C: clinical phenotype at nine years old. Note the midface hypoplasia and the bilateral cleft lip extending across the cheek as a groove to the inner canthus (Tessier cleft number 4. The cleft was more severe on the right side. D-F: facial phenotype at 19 years old. Observe the maxilla sagittal deficiency with a Class III skeletal pattern. G-J: computed tomography 3D reconstructions obtained at age 16. On the right side, observe a wide bone cleft in the frontal maxillary process (arrows). A slight hypoplasia of the frontal maxillary process was observed on the left side. K: an upper airway lateral view demonstrated a normal morphological oropharynx. L: panoramic radiograph at 16 years old showing agenesis of the maxillary lateral incisor (12) and second premolar (15). Alveolar defects (between 11–13).

CHAPTER SIX

TESSIER CLEFT NUMBER 5: THE ORBITO-MAXILLARY CLEFT

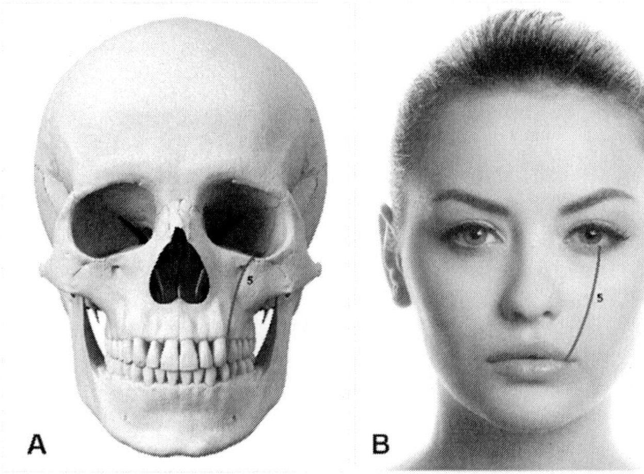

Figure 31 – Localization of Tessier cleft number 5. (A) Bone clefts numbered. (B) Soft tissue clefts numbered. Original artwork by the authors.

Tessier cleft number 5, or orbito-maxillary cleft, is characterized by a median cleft lip that extends to the middle and lateral third of the lower eyelid. Ocular malformations may occur. In bone tissue, the alveolar cleft is located between the canine and premolar regions, extending superiorly through the maxilla until the lower infraorbital rim (lateral to the infraorbital foramen), Figure 31.

References

Cannistrà, C., C. Bontemps, R. Valero, G. Iannetti, and J. P. Barbet. 2006. "Orbitofacial Cleft Number 5: Radiographic, Anatomical and Histologic Study of a 24-Week-Old Fetus." *Plast Reconstr Surg* 118 (7): 1538–42. https://doi.org/ 10.1097/01.prs.0000240818.64018.2a

Da Silva Freitas, R., Alonso N. Shin, J. H. Busato, L. Dal,' 'oglio Tolazzi, and A. R. De Oliveria E Cruz. 2009. "The Tessier Number 5 Facial Cleft: Surgical Strategies and Outcomes in Six Patients." *Cleft Palate Craniofac J* 46 (2): 179–86. https://doi.org/ 10.1597/07-192.1

David, D. J., M. H. Moore, and R. D. Cooter. 1989. "Tessier Clefts Revisited with a Third Dimension." *Cleft Palate J* 26 (3): 184–85.

Racz, C., S. Dakpé, and N. Kadlub. 2018. "Phenotypic Spectrum of Tessier Facial Cleft Number 5." *J Craniomaxillofac Surg* 46 (1): 22–27. https://doi.org/ 10.1016/j.jcms.2017.10.012

Tessier, Paul. 1976. "Anatomical Classification of Facial, Cranio-Facial and Latero-Facial Clefts." *Journal of Maxillofacial Surgery* 4: 69–92. https://doi.org/10.1016/s0301-0503(76)80013-6.

Winters, Ryan. 2016. "Tessier Clefts and Hypertelorism". *Facial Plastic Surgery Clinics of North America* 24 (4): 545–58. https://doi.org/10.1016/j.fsc.2016.06.013.

Tessier cleft number 5

Case 25

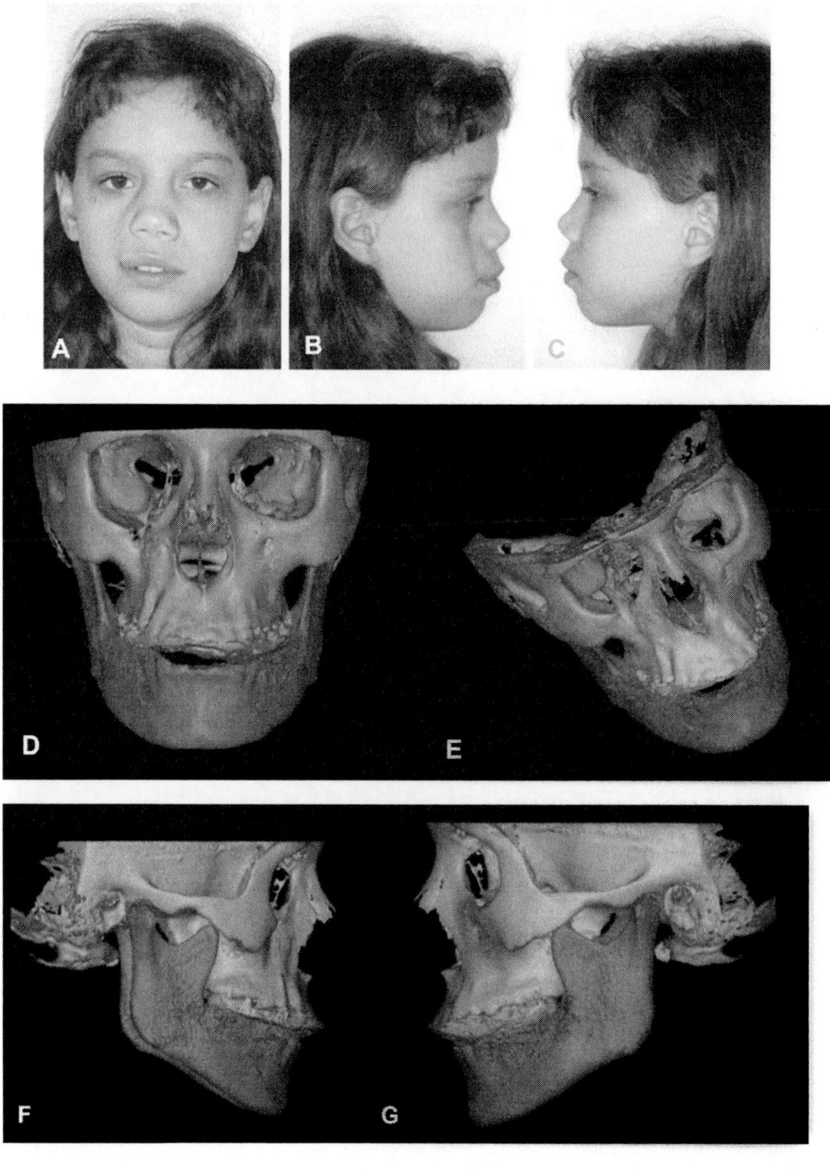

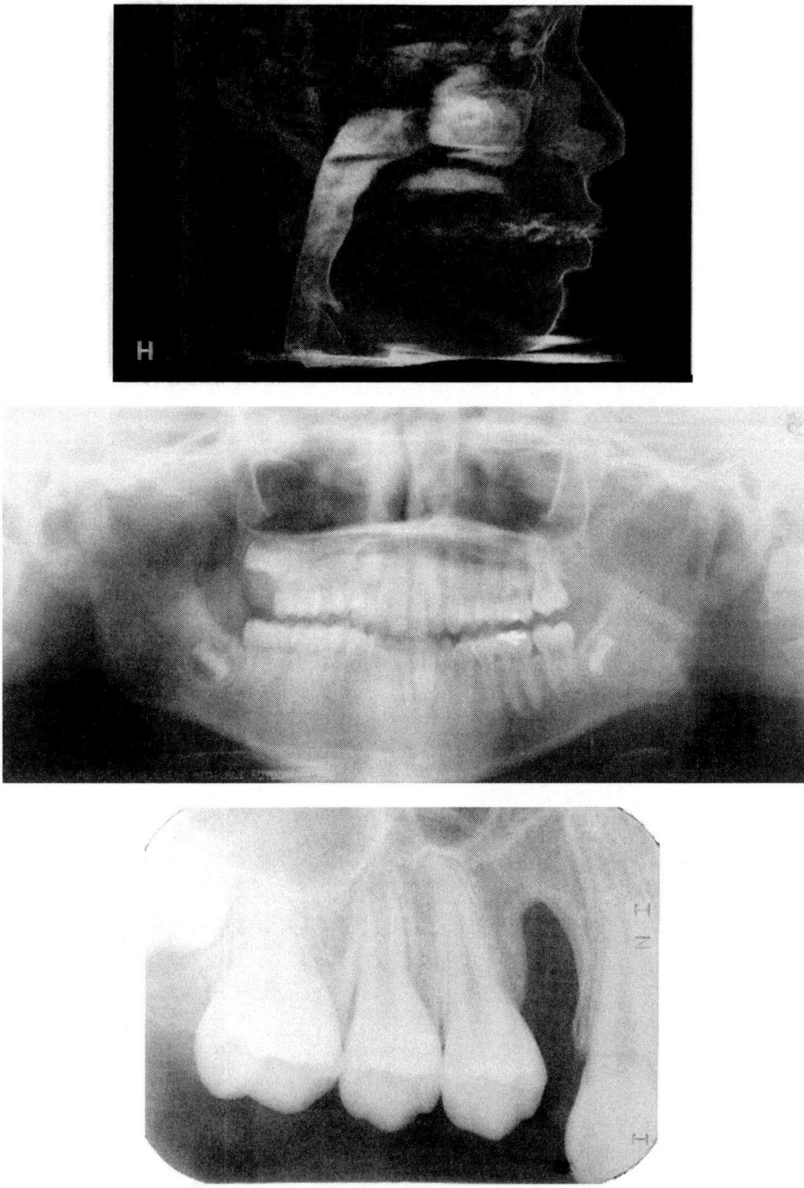

Figure 32 – Female patient with a right Tessier cleft number 5. A-C: Clinical phenotype at nine years old girl. Note the soft tissue, a broad

forehead and a right notch in midface tissue between the eye and the upper lip, just medial to the corner of the mouth. D-G: computed tomography 3D reconstructions obtained at age 16 years old. Note a bone cleft extending from the inferior orbital rim to the premolar region on the right side. H: the upper airway lateral view is normal. I-J: panoramic and periapical radiograph at 12 years old showing no dental anomalies and (J) maxillary alveolar defects between the canine and first premolar (13–14) on the right.

Case 26

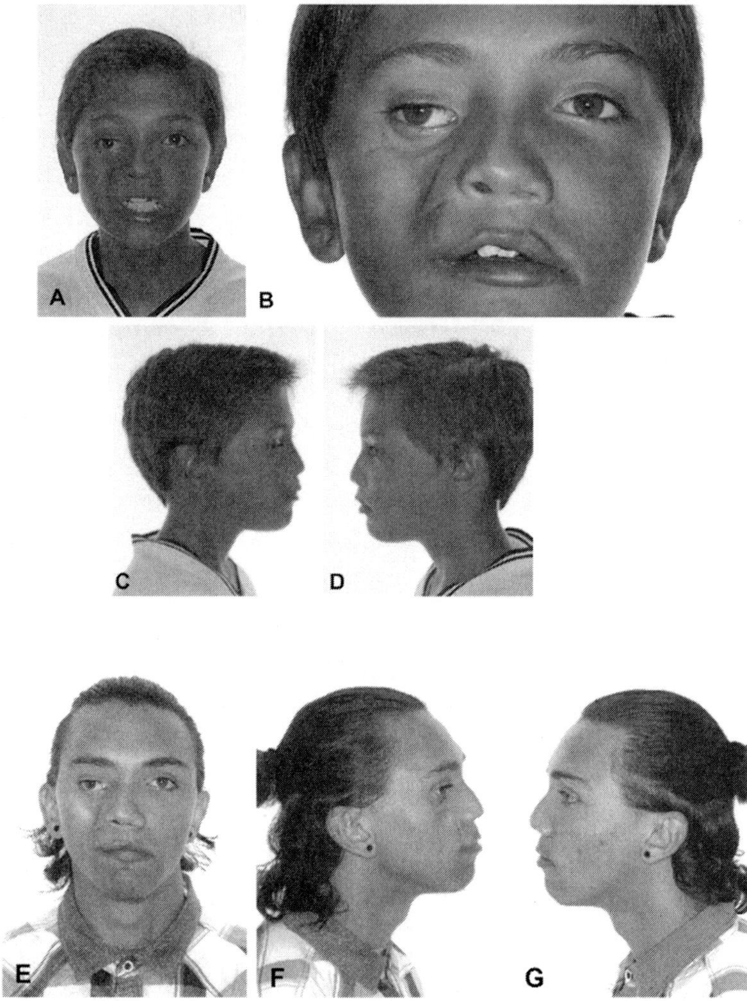

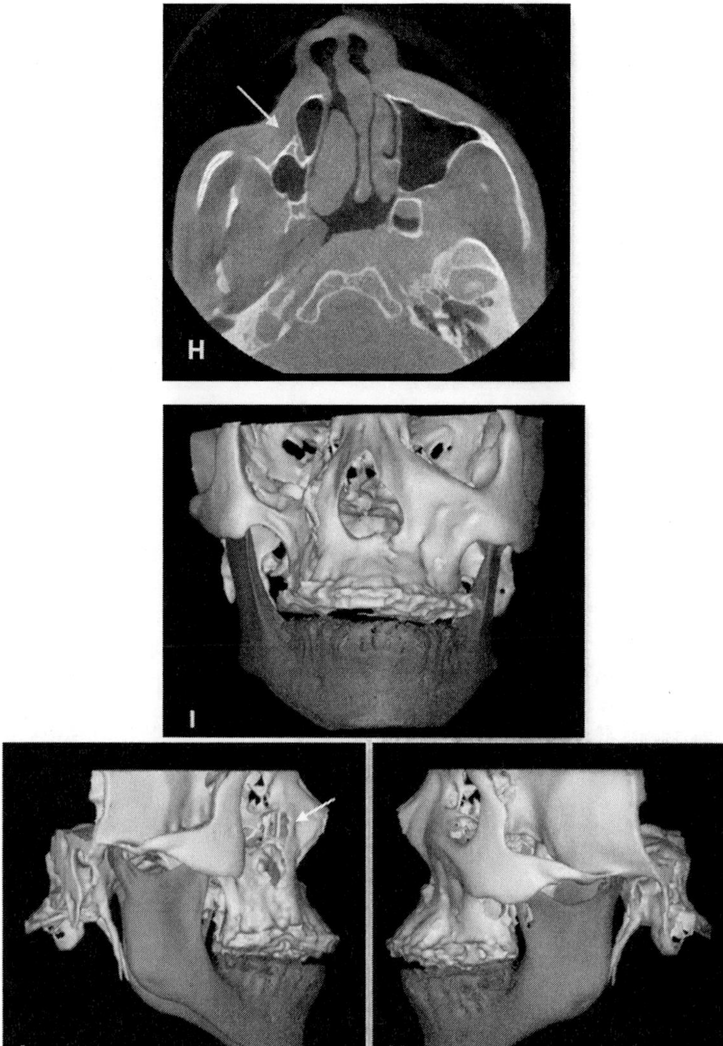
H
I
J
K

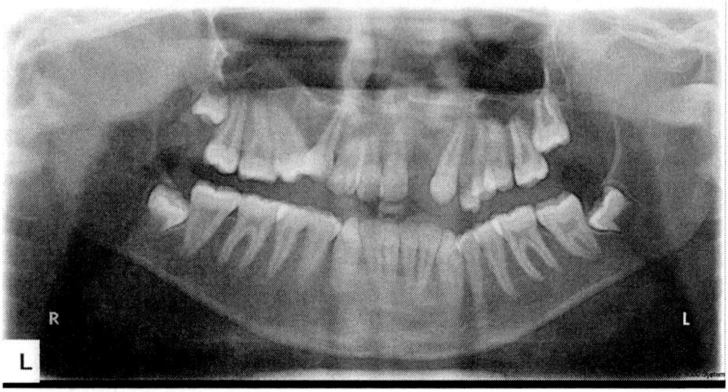

Figure 33– Male patient with a right unilateral Tessier cleft number 5. A-D: clinical phenotype at nine years old. Observe the slight face asymmetry with the right repaired cleft lip and palate on the left. On the right side, the cleft lip started medially to the oral commissure extending across the cheek as a groove to the middle of the lower eyelid (Tessier cleft number 5). E-G: clinical phenotype at 17 years old showing a broad forehead, a lower eyelid and a midface hypoplasia on the right side. G-J: computed tomography taken at 17 years old. Figure H demonstrates an axial section showing the bone failure in the right zygomatic bone, the hypoplastic maxilla and maxillary sinus on the right side and the nasal septum deviation (arrow). In the CT three-dimensional reconstructions (Figures I to K), a groove in the alveolar arch reaching the nasal cavity is apparent on the left side. On the right side, a cleft in the medial orbital rim extending horizontally towards to inner canthus and vertically to the maxillary frontal process, and finishing in the upper region, the alveolar ridge between premolar and molar region is observed (Tessier cleft number 5). In the lateral view (Figure J), note a bone cleft in the frontal process of the maxilla (arrow). The zygomatic bone is hypoplastic on the right side. The zygomatic arch is short and hypoplastic bilaterally. L: panoramic radiograph at 13 years old showing agenesis of the maxillary lateral incisors (22) and alveolar defects between the central incisors and canines (21–23) on the left.

Case 27

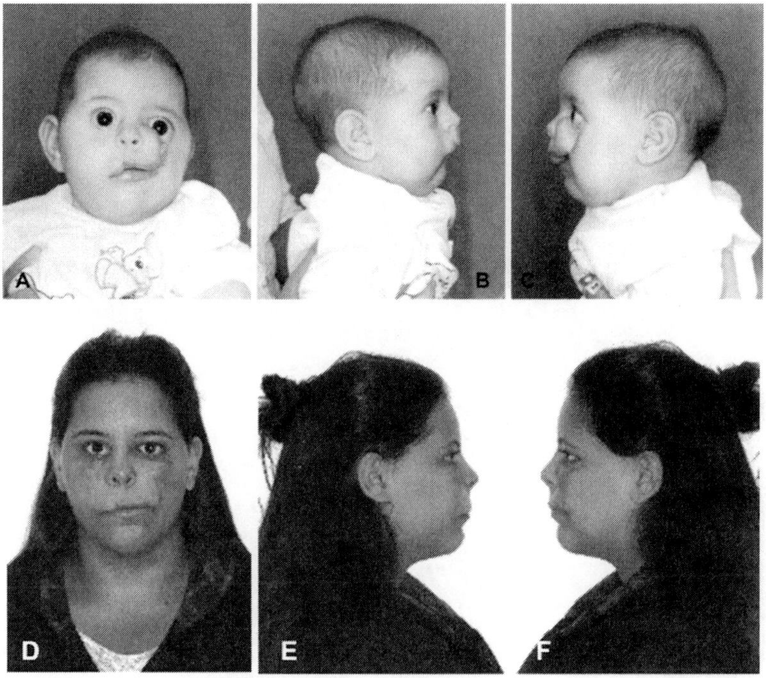

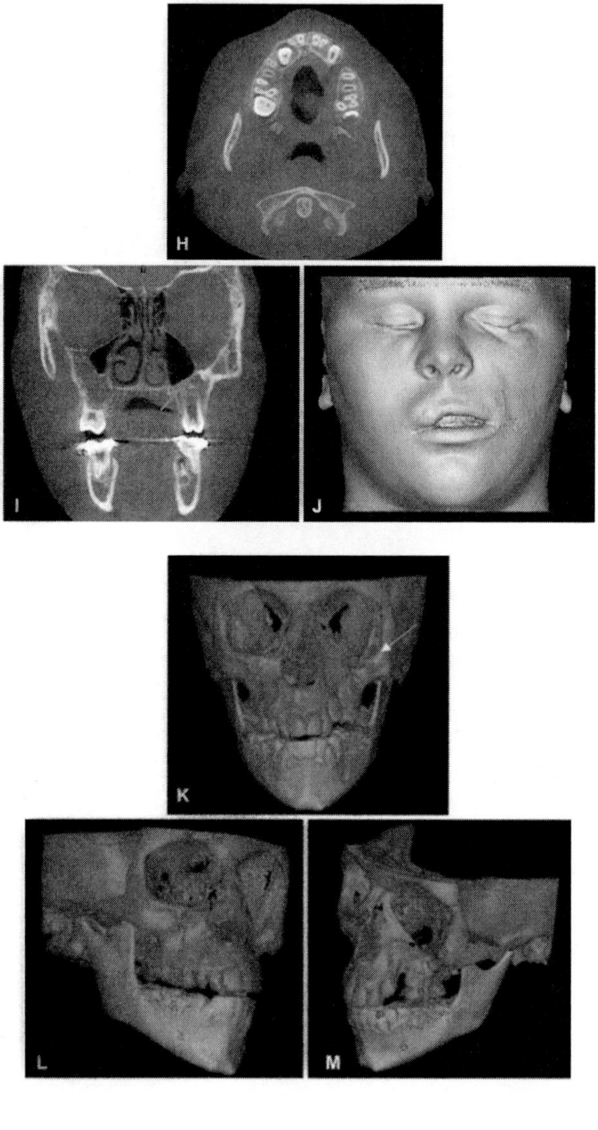
H
I
J
K
L
M

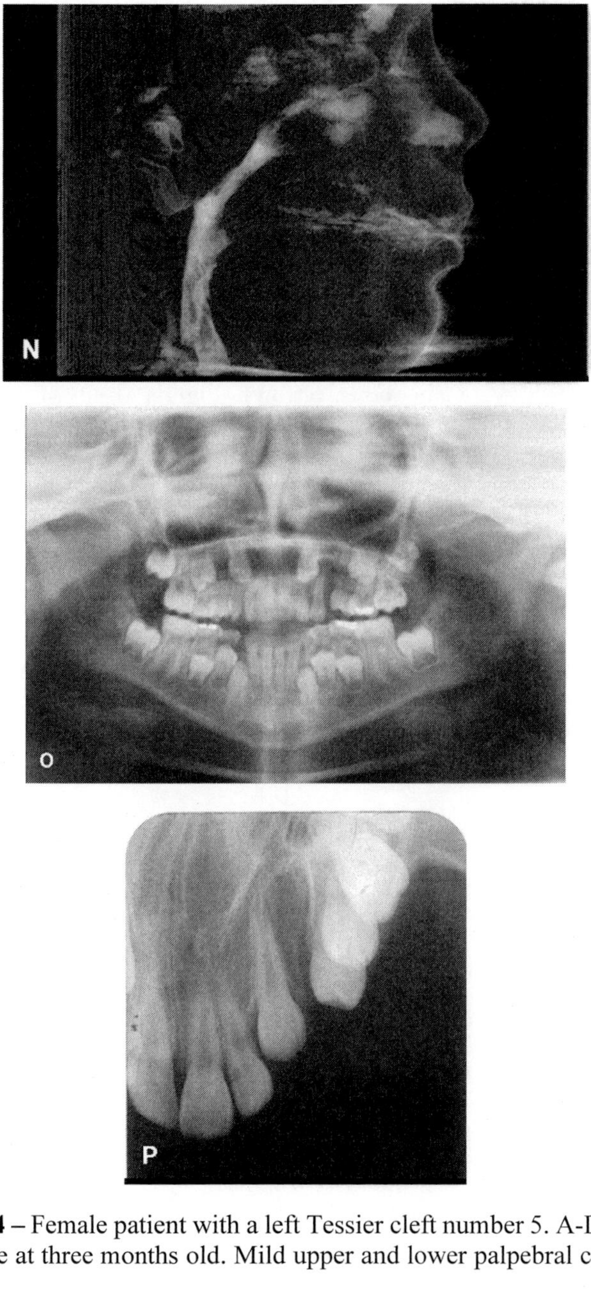

Figure 34 – Female patient with a left Tessier cleft number 5. A-D: clinical phenotype at three months old. Mild upper and lower palpebral colobomas between the inner canthus and lacrimal punctum are observed in the soft tissue. There is a left cleft lip beginning close to the oral commissure, extending across the cheek, and finishing in the medial region of the lower eyelid as a great coloboma that displaces the eyelid (Tessier cleft number 5). Observe a shortening in length between the oral commissure and the lower eyelid on the left and a macrostomia. On the right side, a scar cleft lip extending to the ocular region as a groove is present (Tessier cleft number 4). D-F: facial photographs at 17 years old show facial asymmetry and a shortened nasal length. H-J: computed tomography was taken at ten years old. In figure H an axial section passing at the level of the maxillary alveolar ridge shows the left alveolar cleft in the mesial aspect of the premolar region. Figure I is a coronal section at the level of premolars showing the cleft over the zygomatic bone (arrow). Figures J to M are CT 3D reconstructions. Figure J displays the soft tissue deficiency along both margins of the orbital cleft. In the bone tissue (Figures K to M), observe the right side midfacial hypoplasia and a notch in the infraorbital rim (mild Tessier number four). On the left side, a wide alveolar cleft starts in the premolar region and extends to the maxillary sinus until the infraorbital rim is present (Tessier cleft number 5). Figure N, the upper airway lateral view is normal. O-P: panoramic and periapical radiograph at nine years old showing absence of dental anomalies and (P) showing maxillary alveolar defect between the canine and first premolar (23-24) on the left.

Case 28

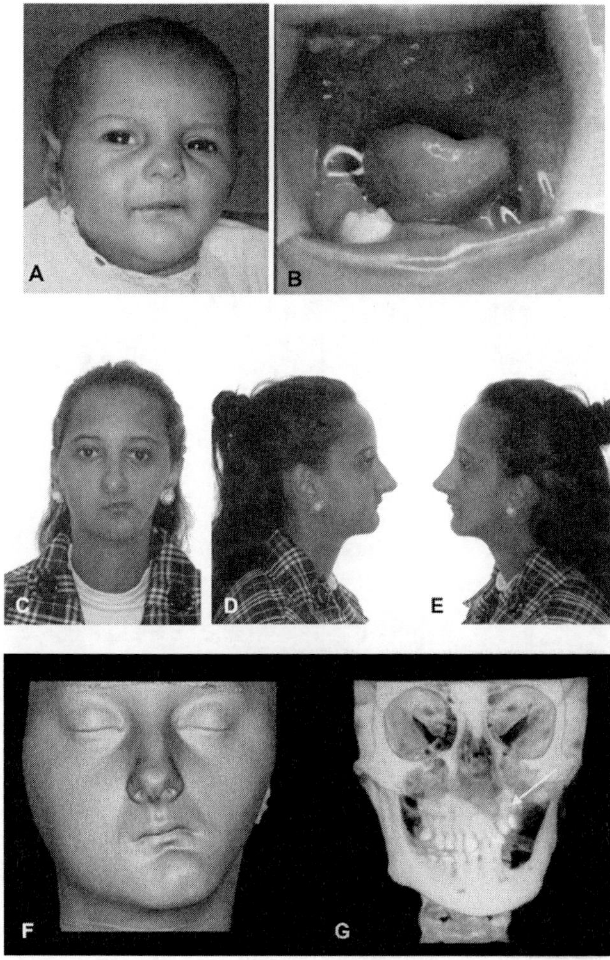

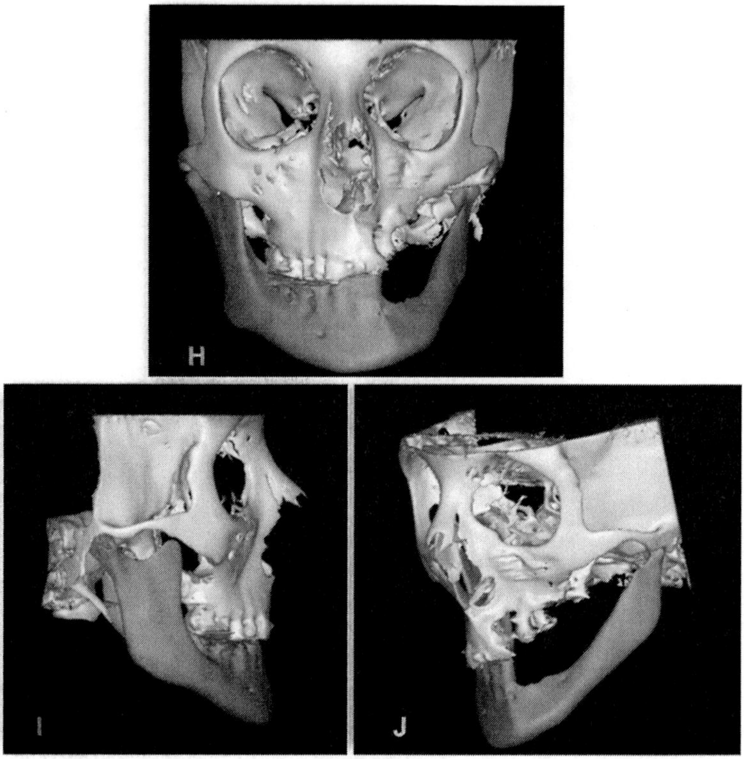

Figure 35 – Female patient with a left Tessier cleft number 5. A-B: clinical phenotype at three months old. Observe the microglossia and mild asymmetry in the lower face. Intraorally, a small tongue with hypoplasia of the mandibular alveolar ridge on the left side is noted. C-E: clinical phenotype at 19 years old showing a worsening of the facial asymmetry, a midface hypoplasia, a narrow nasal base, a short philtrum, a microstomia and a micrognathia. F-J: computed tomography taken at 26 years old. Figure F shows a soft tissue three-dimensional reconstruction of the severe mandibular asymmetry. Figure G is a translucent 3D reconstruction showing the left upper alveolar cleft in the premolar region (arrow), representing the Tessier cleft number 5. An abnormal mandibular bone with multiple dental agenesis is observed on the left side. Figures H to J reveal, on the left side, an incomplete Tessier cleft number 5 in the bone tissue extending from the maxillary premolar region to the infraorbital rim as a notch associated with severe maxillary hypoplasia. A significant mandibular body and ramus hypoplasia on the left side with agenesis, the

coronoid process and condylar hypoplasia is observed. Multiple tooth agenesis is present in the maxillary arch (21, 22, 23, 26, 27 and 28) and mandibular arch (48, 41, 31, 32, 33, 34, 35, 36, 37 and 38).

CHAPTER SEVEN

TESSIER CLEFT NUMBER 6: THE MAXILLARY-ZYGOMATIC CLEFT

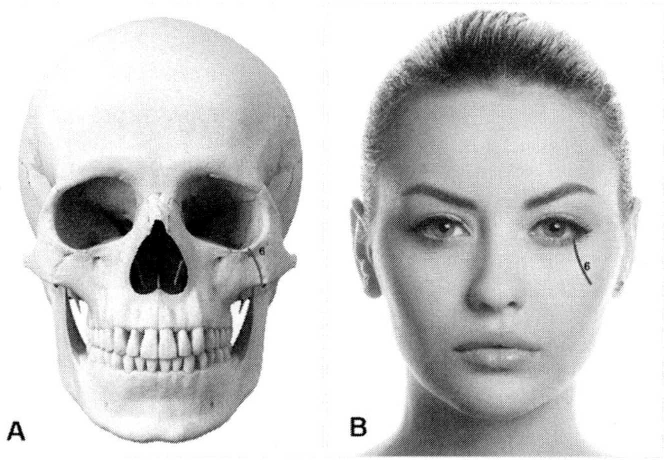

Figure 36 – Localization of Tessier cleft number 6. (A) Bone clefts numbered. (B) Soft tissue clefts numbered. Original artwork by the authors.

Tessier cleft number 6, or the zygomaticomaxillary cleft, is characterized in the soft tissue by a groove in the middle third of the lower eyelid with the presence of coloboma extending downward through the cheek to the labial commissure. The cleft is between the maxilla and the zygomatic bone, opening the infraorbital lower border (Figure 36). Tessier cleft number 6 is frequently observed in Treacher Collins syndrome.

References

Cobb, A. R., B. Green, and D. Gill. 2014. "The Surgical Management of Treacher Collins Syndrome." *Br J Oral Maxillofac Surg* 52 (7): 581–89. https://doi.org/ 10.1016/j.bjoms.2014.02.007.

David, D. J., M. H. Moore, and R. D. Cooter. 1989. "Tessier Clefts Revisited with a Third Dimension." *Cleft Palate J* 26 (3): 184–85.

Fijałkowska, M., and B. Antoszewski. 2015. "Rare Facial Clefts." *Pol Przegl Chir* 87 (8): 389–94. https://doi.org/ 10.1515/pjs-2015-0077.

Tessier, Paul. 1976. "Anatomical Classification of Facial, Cranio-Facial and Latero-Facial Clefts." *Journal of Maxillofacial Surgery* 4: 69–92. https://doi.org/10.1016/s0301-0503(76)80013-6.

Winters, Ryan. 2016. "Tessier Clefts and Hypertelorism". *Facial Plastic Surgery Clinics of North America* 24 (4): 545–58. https://doi.org/10.1016/j.fsc.2016.06.013.

Tessier cleft number 6

Case 29

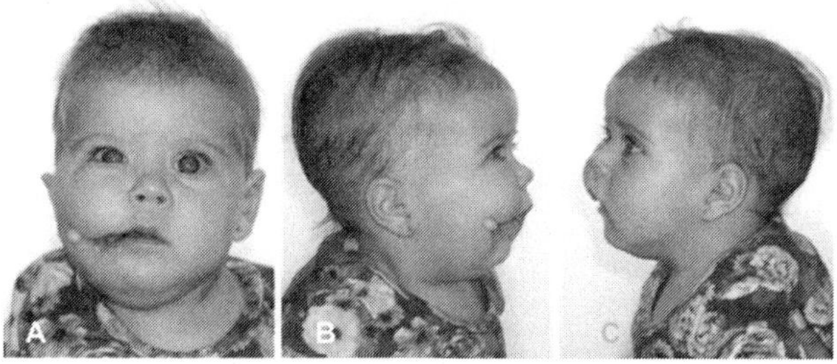

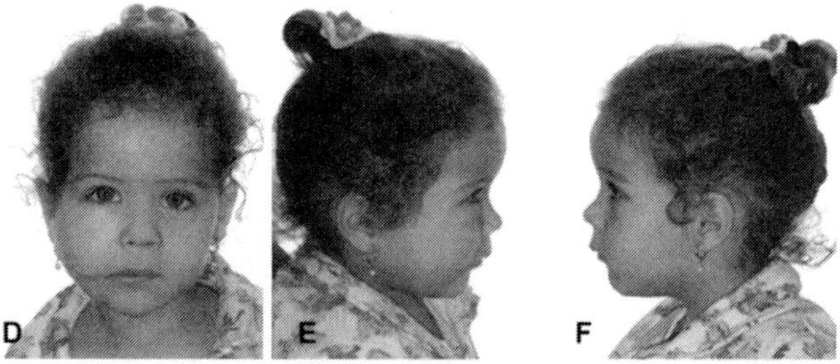

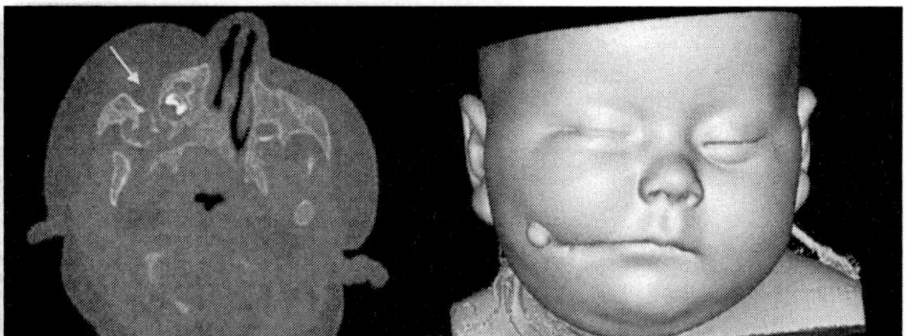

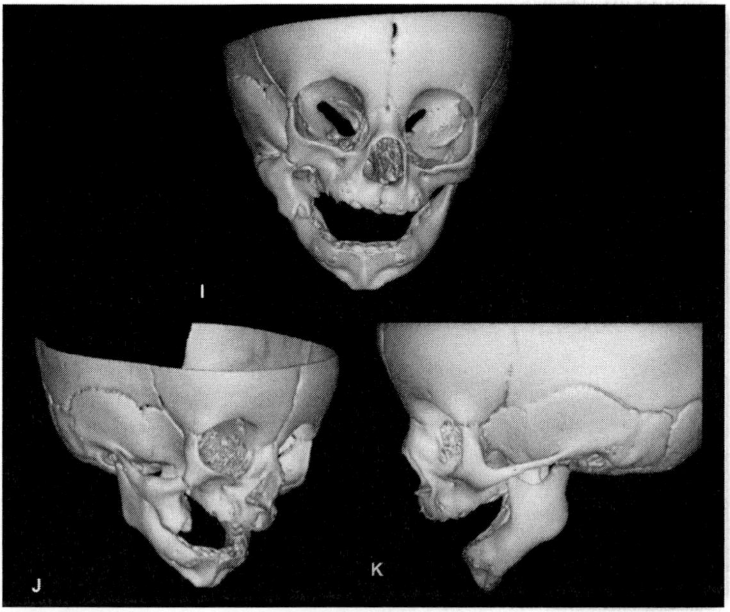

Figure 37– Female patient with a mild right Tessier cleft number 6. A-C: Clinical phenotype at five months old. Observe the soft tissue macrostomia on the right side with the mild cleft extending from the oral commissure with a mild furrow across the cheek to the lateral canthus lower eyelid (Tessier cleft number 6). The right oral commissure cleft extends laterally towards the preauricular region to the middle cheek finishing in a large skin tag (incomplete Tessier cleft number 7). D-F: clinical phenotype at 23 months old demonstrating a facial asymmetry at the level of midface and ocular regions. G-K: computed tomography exams taken at four months old. Figure G is an axial section showing the zygomatic cleft with a lateral accessory maxilla and a nasal septum deviation. Figure H is a soft tissue reconstruction showing a slight facial asymmetry, a mild notch in the right outer canthus, the macrostomia and the skin tag. Figures I to K reveal the hard tissue segmentation demonstrating a wide right cleft in the zygomatic bone (arrow) with the abnormal structure of the zygomatic arch and an atopic vertical growth of the maxilla, resembling an accessory maxilla which is commonly associated with Tessier cleft number 7.

Case 30

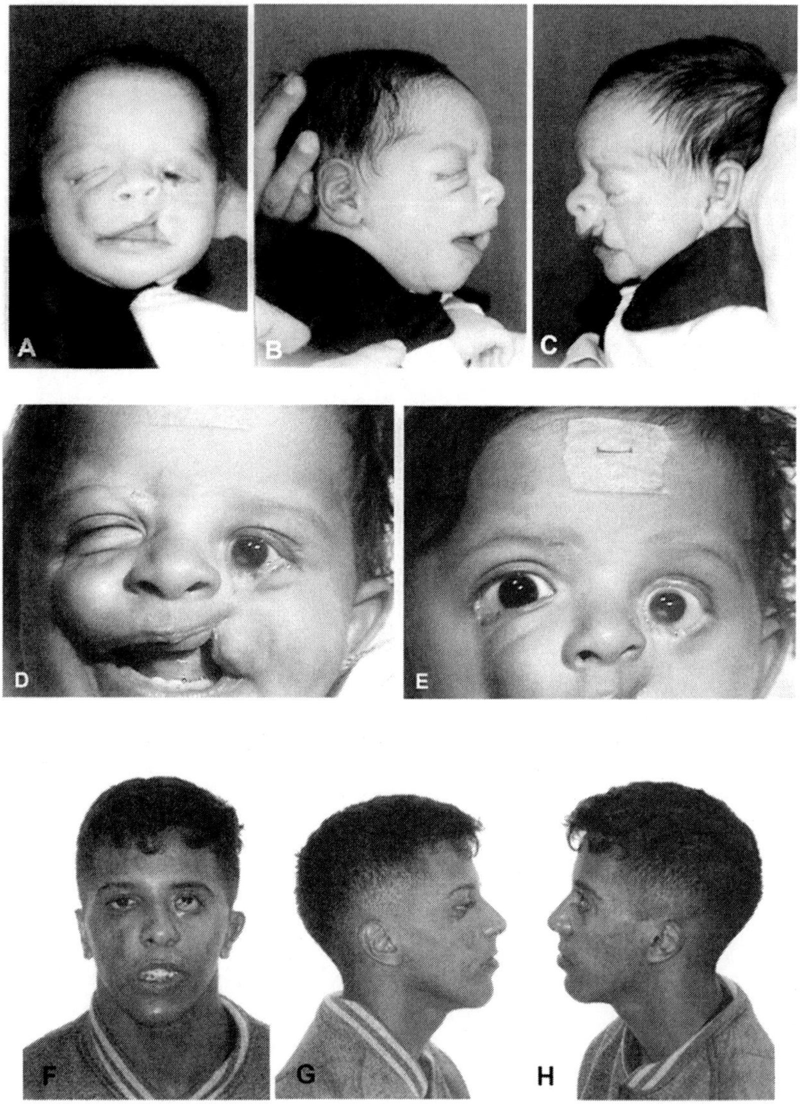

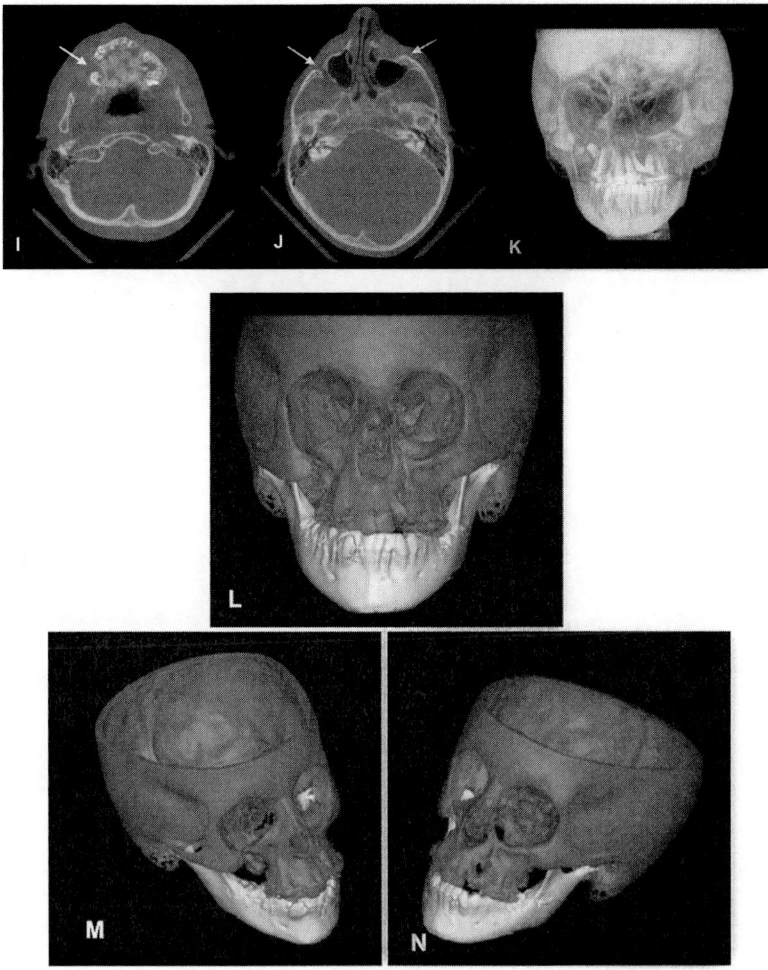
I
J
K
L
M
N

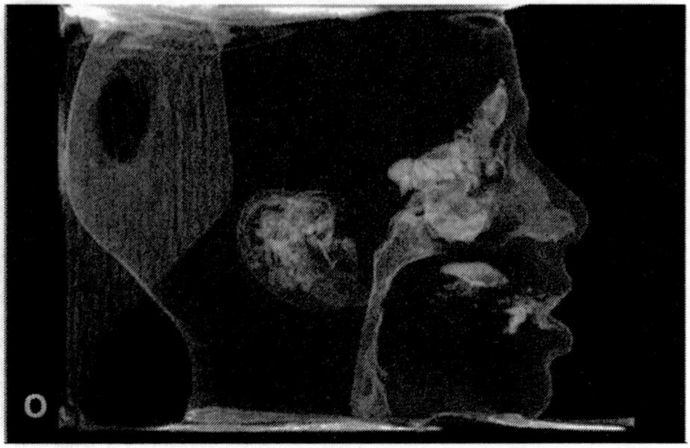

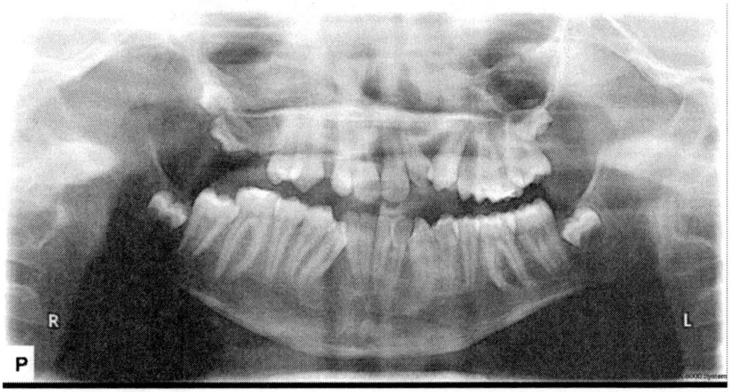

Figure 38 – Male patient with a right Tessier Cleft number 6. A-C: clinical phenotype at 12 days old. D-E: facial photographs at seven months old. Observe the broad forehead, a wide right coloboma in the lower eyelid margin extending as a notch across the cheek until the right oral commissure (Tessier cleft number 6). On the left side, a cleft lip extends across the cheek until the coloboma in the medial lower eyelid (Tessier cleft number 5) with white tissue over the ocular globe in the left eye. F-H: clinical phenotype at 16 years old showing slight facial asymmetry. I-O: computed tomography images taken at 11 years old. Figure I is an axial section at the level of the maxillary alveolar ridge demonstrating the right cleft in the posterior region of the maxilla. Figure J is an axial section at the level of the nasal cavity revealing the bone cleft in the zygomatic bone (arrow) and the nasal septum deviation. Figure K is a translucent 3D reconstruction showing the bilateral cleft in the alveolar arch (Tessier cleft number 6 on the right side and Tessier number 5 on the left). Figures L to N 3D are three-dimensional hard tissue

segmentation showing, on the right side, a Tessier cleft number 6 present in bone tissue in the zygomaticomaxillary region with a normal zygomatic arch. On the left side, note a Tessier cleft number 5 starting at the maxillary alveolar region, crossing the hypoplastic maxilla body and finishing near the lower infraorbital rim. O: The lateral airway view demonstrates a narrow pharynx. P: panoramic radiograph at 12 years old showing alveolar defects of maxillary first premolar (distal 14), agenesis of the maxillary second premolar and first molar (15–16) and alveolar defects between the maxillary lateral incisor and canine tooth (22–23).

CHAPTER EIGHT

TESSIER CLEFT NUMBER 7: THE TEMPOROZYGOMATIC CLEFT (ALSO CALLED THE LATERAL CLEFT)

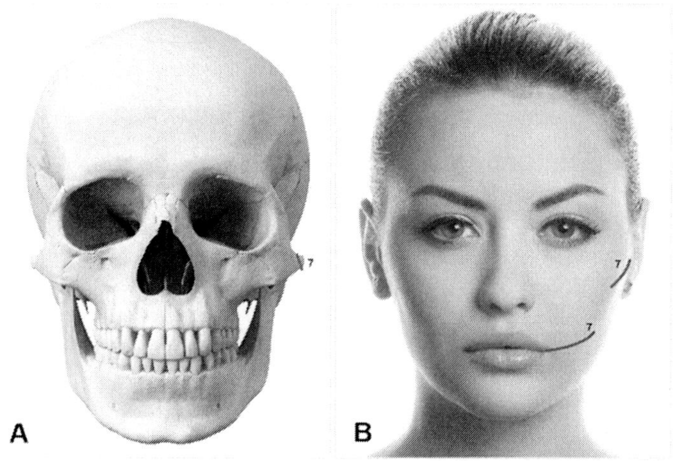

Figure 39 – Localization of Tessier cleft number 7. (A) Bone clefts numbered. (B) Soft tissue clefts numbered. Original artwork by the authors.

Tessier cleft number 7, also known as a temporozygomatic facial cleft or transverse facial cleft, is represented by a cleft in the labial commissure resulting in soft tissue macrostomia, commonly observed in cases of hemifacial microsomia, oculoauriculovertebral spectrum, Nager syndrome, Treacher Collins syndrome and amniotic band sequence. At the level of bone tissue, cleft number 7 affects the temporozygomatic region with the absence of the zygomatic arch or the presence of a cleft in the arch (Figure 39). Tessier cleft number 7 may be associated with accessory maxillae and mandibular anomalies involving the ascending mandibular ramus, the condyle and the coronoid process. In soft tissue, the macrostomia may appear by itself or together with other deformities and may cause difficulties in facial expressions, mastication and speech.

References

Borzabadi-Farahani, A., S. L. Yen, C. Francis, P. A. Lara-Sanchez, and J. Hammoudeh. 2013. "A Rare Case of Accessory Maxilla and Bilateral Tessier No. 7 Clefts, a 10-Year Follow-Up." *J Craniomaxillofac Surg* 41 (6): 527–31. https://doi.org/ 10.1016/j.jcms.2012.11.019

Cobb, A. R., B. Green, and D. Gill. 2014. "The Surgical Management of Treacher Collins Syndrome." *Br J Oral Maxillofac Surg* 52 (7): 581–89. https://doi.org/ 10.1016/j.bjoms.2014.02.007

David, D. J., M. H. Moore, and R. D. Cooter. 1989. "Tessier Clefts Revisited with a Third Dimension." *Cleft Palate J* 26 (3): 184–85.

Hassanpour, S. E., F. H. Shirazi, and F. Karim. 2018. "Lateral Lower Lip Cleft: A Report of a Rare Craniofacial Cleft in a Child." *J Craniofac Surg* 29 (7): e656–58. https://doi.org/ 10.1097/SCS.0000000000004669

Hennekam, Raoul, Judith E. Allanson, and Ian Krantz. 2010. *Gorlin's Syndromes of the Head and Neck*. 5th ed. New York, NY: Oxford University Press.

Hou, M., C. Liu, J. Wang, L. Zhang, and Q. Gao. 2015. "Lateral or Oblique Facial Clefts Associated with Accessory Maxillae: Review of the Literature and Report of a Case." *J Craniomaxillofac Surg* 43 (5): 585–92. https://doi.org/ 10.1016/j.jcms.2015.02.008

Tessier, Paul. 1976. "Anatomical Classification of Facial, Cranio-Facial and Latero-Facial Clefts." *Journal of Maxillofacial Surgery* 4: 69–92. https://doi.org/10.1016/s0301-0503(76)80013-6.

Ryu, Jeong Yeop, Pil Seon Eo, Lulu Tian, Joon Seok Lee, Jeong Woo Lee, Kang Young Choi, Jung Dug Yang, Ho Yun Chung and Byung Chae Cho. 2019. "Surgical Correction for Tessier Number 7 Craniofacial Cleft Using a Medially Overcorrected Design." *Archives of Plastic Surgery* 46 (01): 16–22. https://doi.org/10.5999/aps.2018.01193.

Case 31

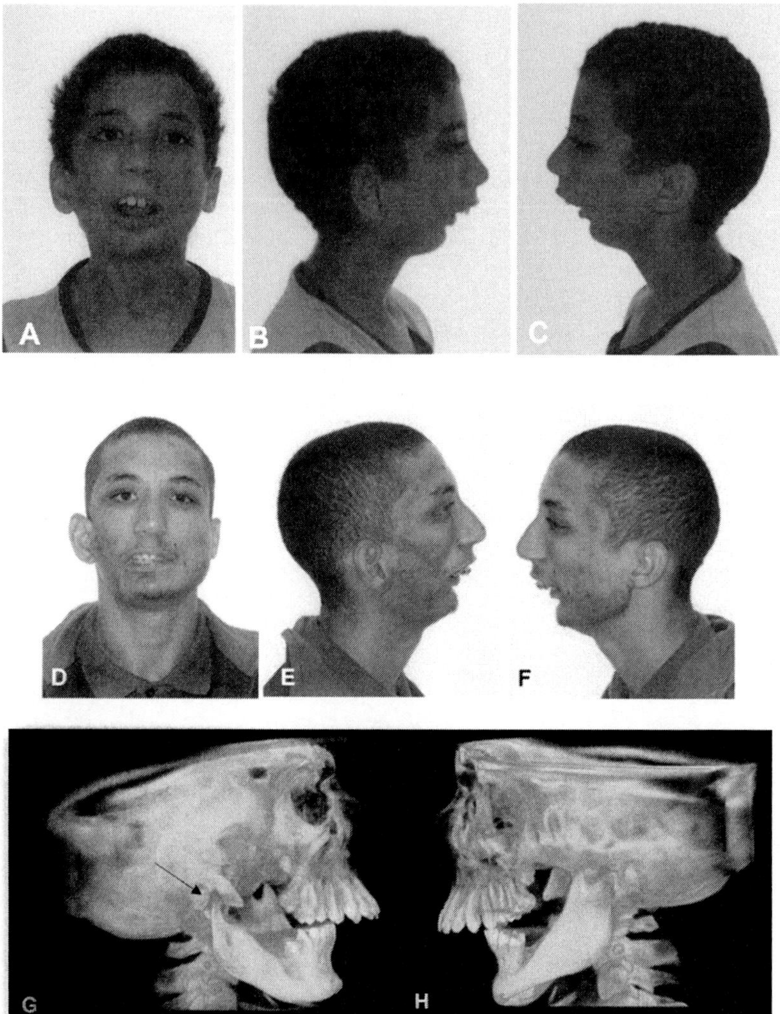

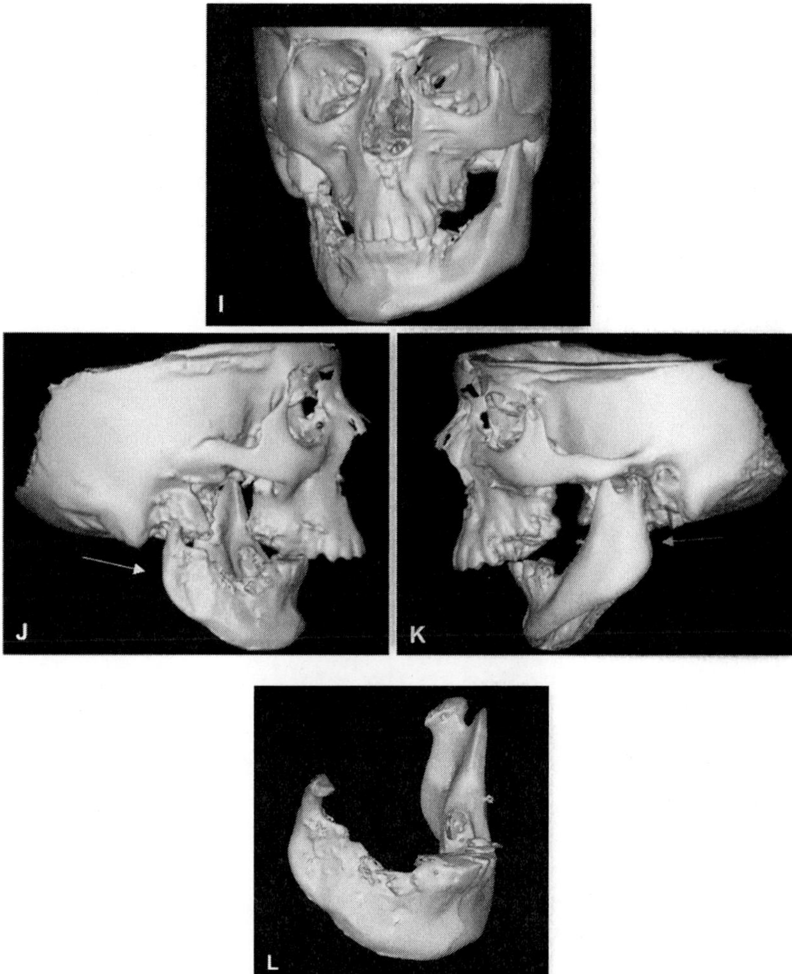

Figure 40– Male patient with a bilateral Tessier cleft number 7. A-C: clinical phenotype at ten years old. Note the facial asymmetry, the macrostomia with a repaired right lateral cleft and scar extending to the preauricular region, severe micrognathia and low-set ears. D-F: clinical phenotype at 17 years old showing a worsening of the facial asymmetry, a maxilla protruding and a severe mandibular micrognathia moderate protrusion of the upper incisors, resulting in a severe increase in the horizontal overlap. G-K: computed tomography images taken at 11 years

old. Figures G and H show translucent 3D reconstructions showing a protruded maxilla, a hypoplastic zygoma and a morphologically abnormal and small mandible. Figures I to L are hard tissue CT segmentation displaying the facial asymmetry, a short zygomatic arch with atopic insertion on the right side. A bony segment in the temporomandibular region that projects vertically toward the mandibular ramus is observed on the right side. The mandible is retrognathic and asymmetric, displaying a deformity of both mandibular ramus (arrow). On the right side, observe the condyle hypoplasia and the agenesis of the coronoid process and glenoid fossa.

Case 32

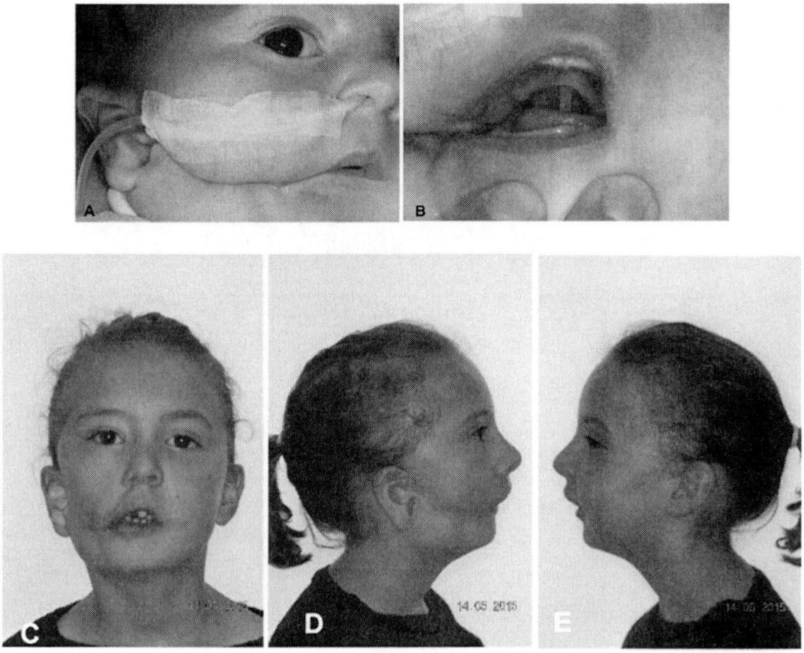

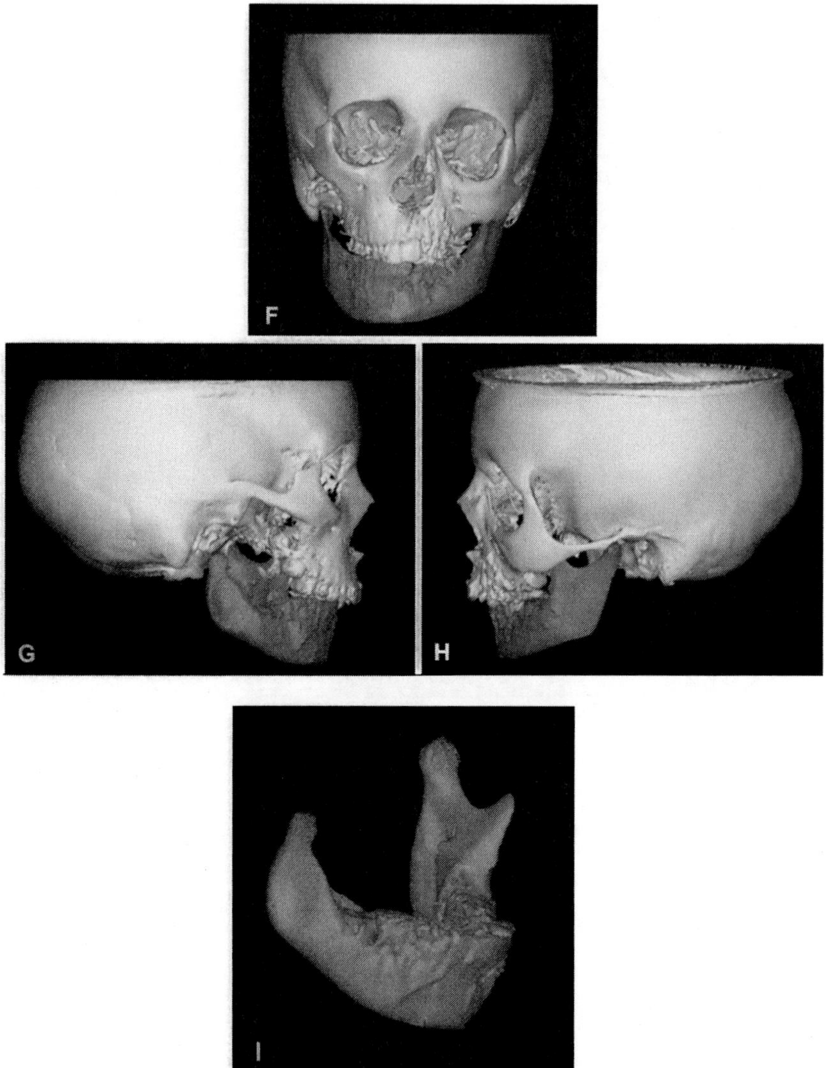
F
G
H
I

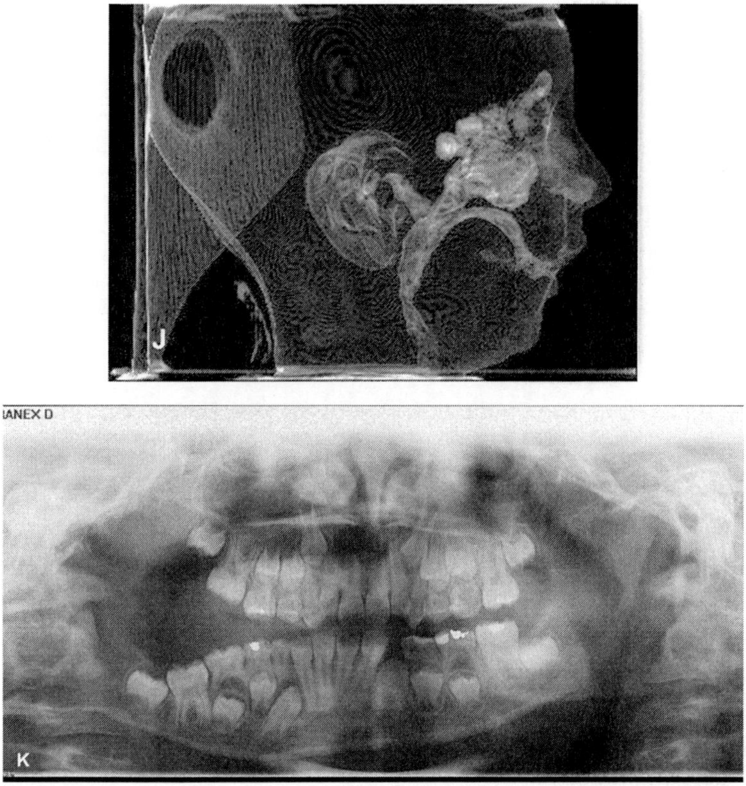

Figure 41 – Female patient with a right Tessier cleft number 7 associated with Robin sequence. A-B: clinical phenotype at two months old. Observe the right lateral cleft originating at the oral commissure and extending toward the preauricular region affecting the tragus and finishing in the auricular concha (Tessier cleft number 7). Figure B shows a small oral aperture or narrow mouth, a complete lateral cleft (Tessier cleft number 7), a U-shaped cleft palate and a posteriorly displaced tongue. C-E: clinical phenotype at six years old showing the repaired lateral cleft, a facial asymmetry, a micrognathia and an abnormal right ear. F-H: computed tomography 3D-reconstructions obtained at age 7. Note the facial asymmetry, the short and upslanting zygomatic arch on the right side, a thin zygomatic arch on the left side, and the absence of the right glenoid fossa. I: the mandible showed severe hypoplasia with a malformed right ramus and condyle and agenesis of the coronoid process on the same side. J: the lateral view of the upper airway view demonstrates a narrow oropharynx. K: panoramic radiograph at eight years old showing the absence of dental anomalies.

Case 33

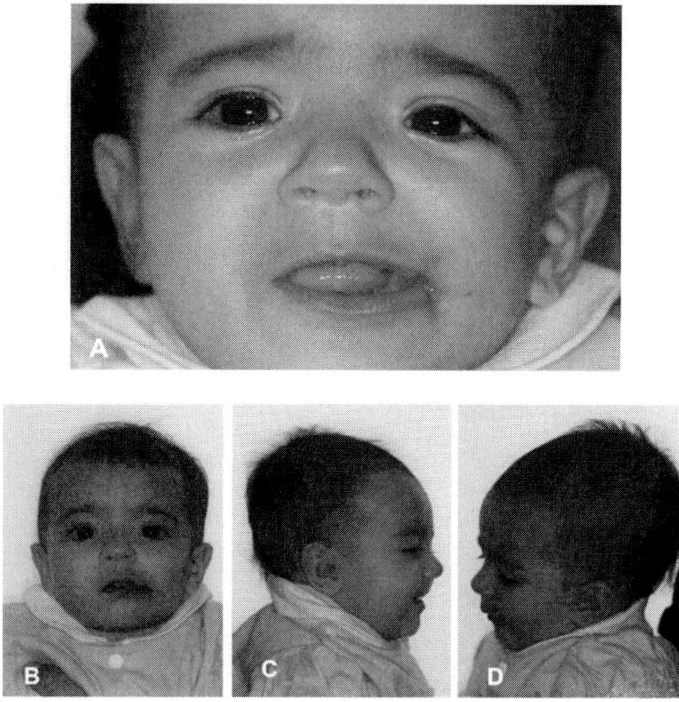

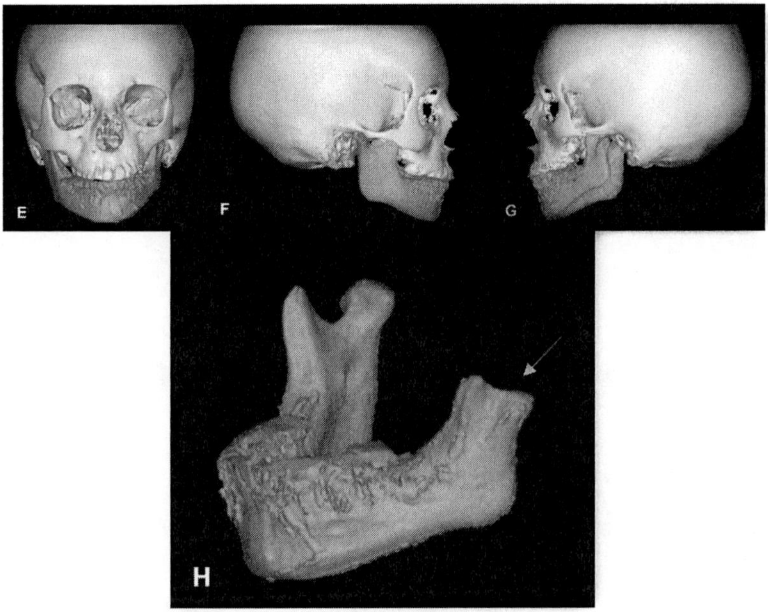

Figure 42– Female patient with a left Tessier cleft number 7. A-D: clinical phenotype at five months old. Note the left lateral facial cleft causing just a mild macrostomia or widened oral commissure. E-H: computed tomography 3D-reconstructions obtained at eight years old. Note a slight mandibular asymmetry with a short left mandibular ramus with agenesis of the condyle and coronoid processes.

Case 34

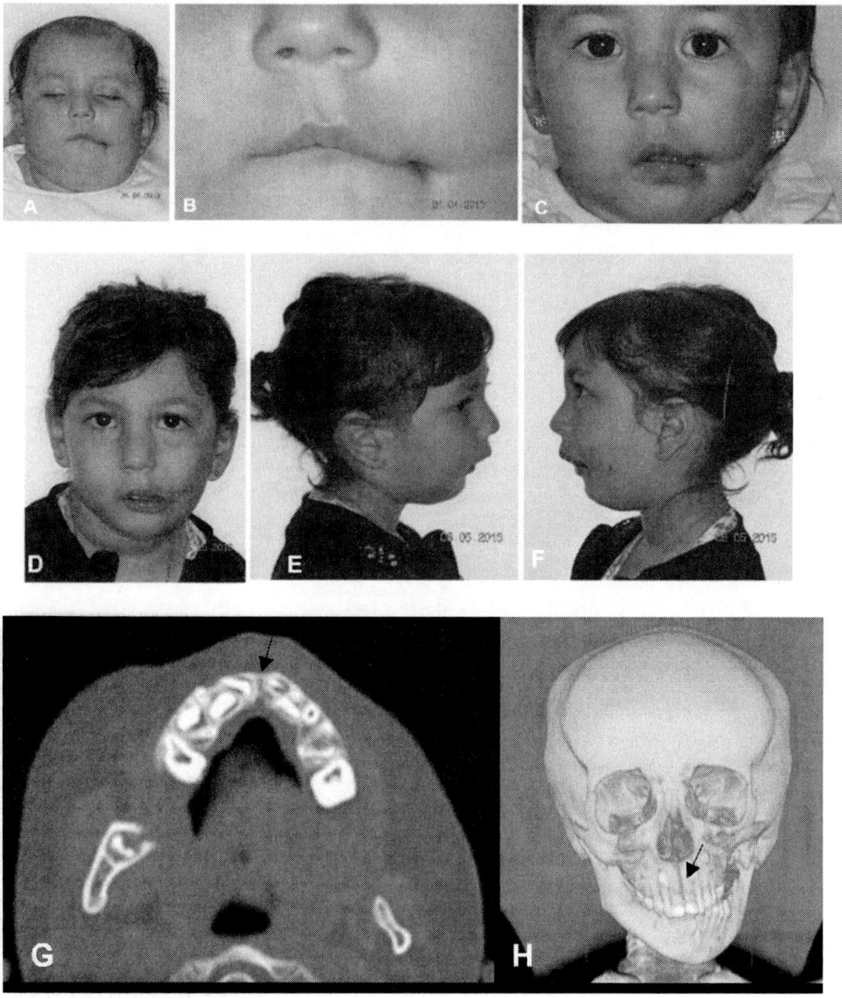

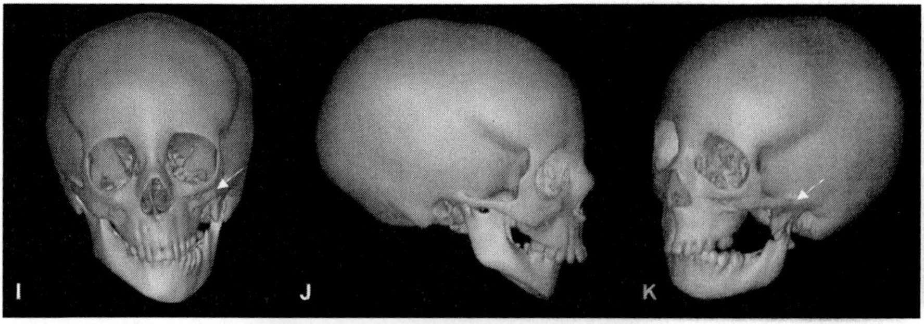

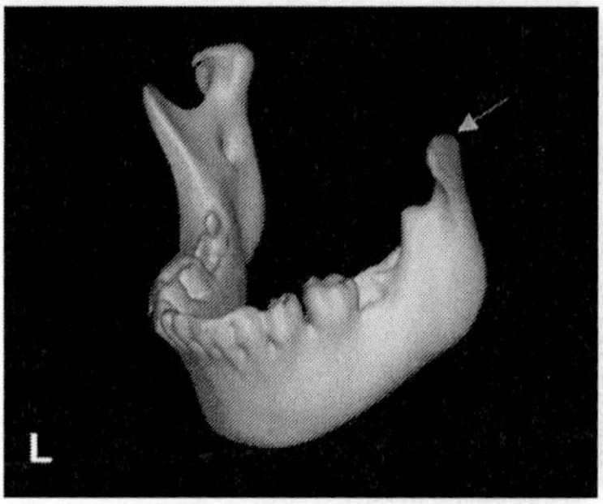

Figure 43–Female patient with a left Tessier cleft number 7. A-C: clinical phenotype at nine and 11 months old (C). Observe the small oral aperture or narrow mouth, a short lateral facial cleft on the left side causing a macrostomia (Tessier cleft number 7) with a normal red-lip mucosal line on the right side. The left lateral cleft extended as a mild notch across the cheek toward the outer eye canthus (mild Tessier cleft number 6). D-F: facial photographs at two and a half years old showing a repaired cleft and a mandibular asymmetry. G-H: computed tomography exam taken at age four. Figure G shows an axial section revealing the left cleft in the maxilla. Figure H is a translucent 3D reconstruction showing the midline alveolar cleft (arrow) as a mild Tessier cleft number 0. Figure I demonstrates a midface hypoplasia, a bone failure just below the left lower infraorbital rim in both the maxilla and the zygomatic bone (arrow). Figures J and K; note that the left zygomatic arch is short. In the temporal portion of the left zygomatic arch, an accessory bone outgrowth toward the inferior and posterior is observed on the left. The mandible is asymmetric, displaying a short mandibular ramus on the left side, a hypoplastic condyle and an absent coronoid process (Figures K and L).

Case 35

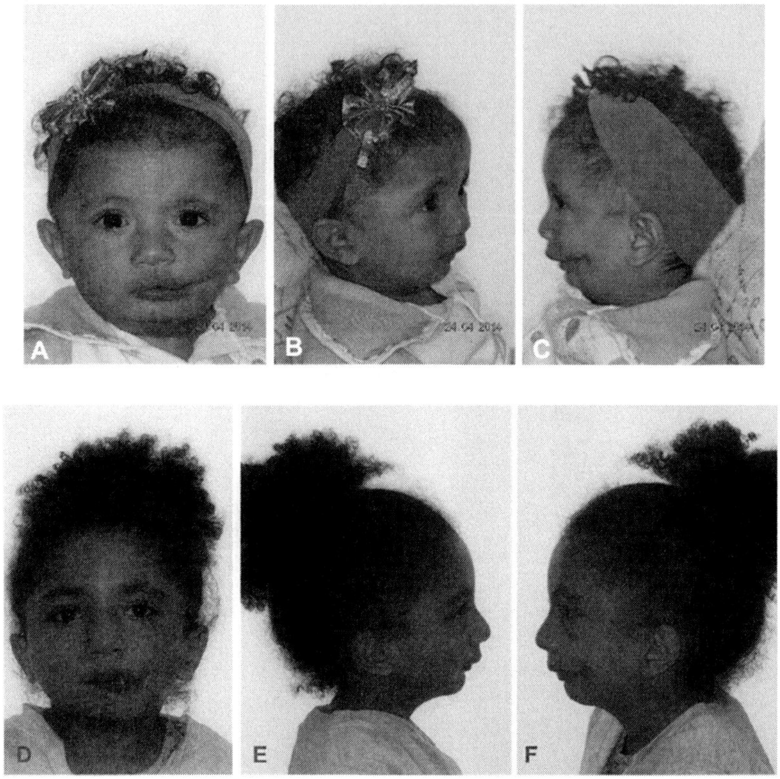

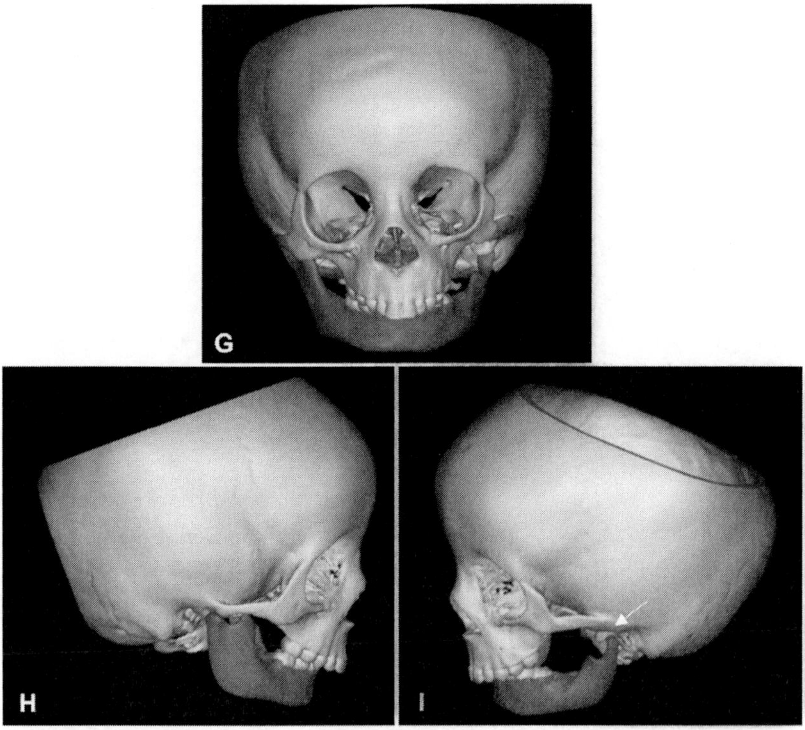

Figure 44 – Female patient with a left Tessier cleft number 7. A-C: clinical phenotype at nine months old. Note an incomplete lateral cleft and macrostomia on the left side. A micrognathia was also present. D-F: facial photographs at six years old showing a repaired lateral cleft (Tessier cleft number 7). G-I: computed tomography 3D images obtained at age three. Note the severe hypoplasia of the left mandibular ramus associated with condylar hypoplasia and agenesis of the coronoid process. There is little additional bone structure fixed to the underlying zygomatic arch on the left side (arrow).

Case 36

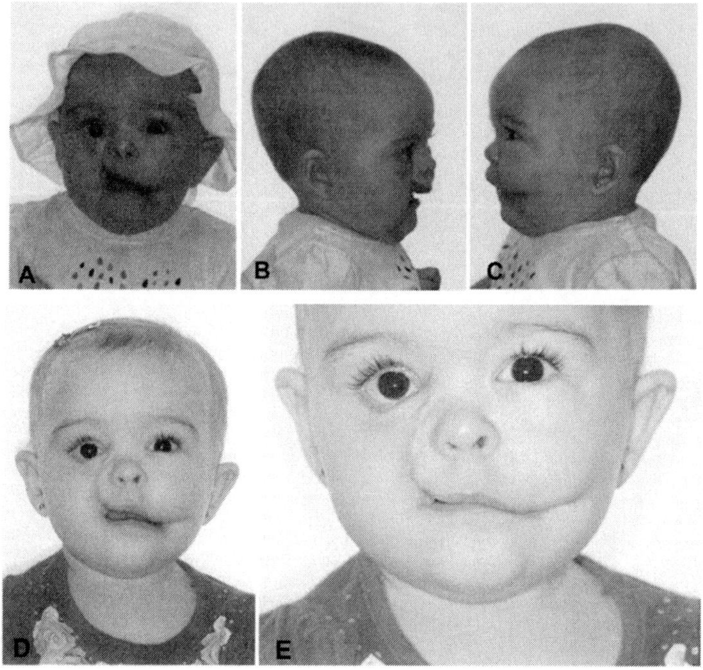

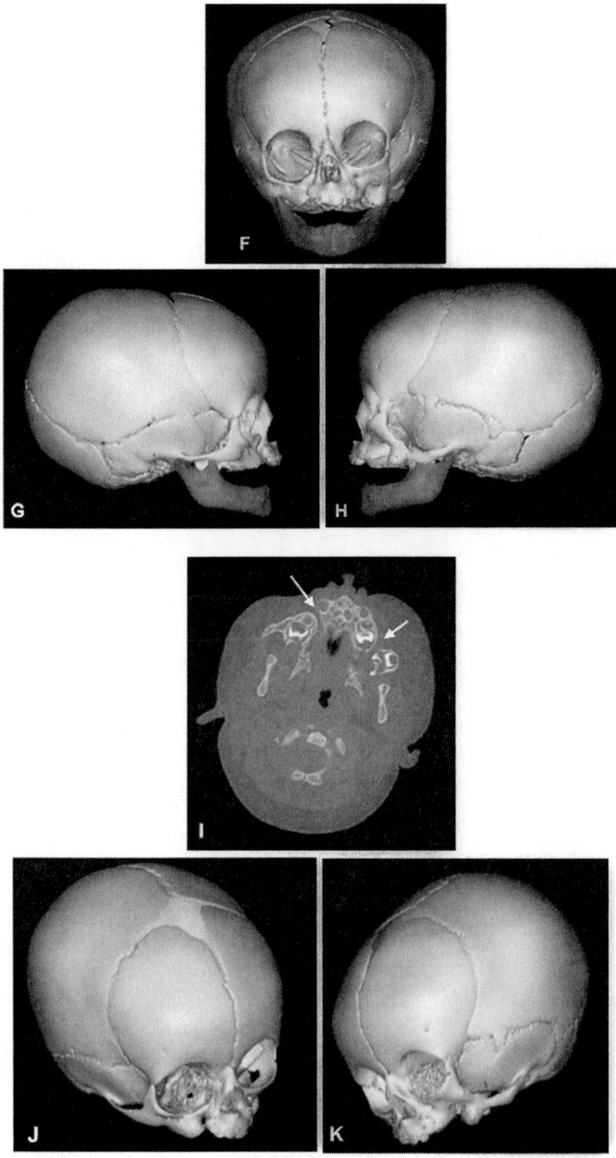

Figure 45 – Female patient with a left Tessier cleft number 7 associated with a right Tessier cleft number 4. A-C: clinical phenotype at nine months old. Note the left incomplete lateral cleft with macrostomia (Tessier cleft

number 7). On the right side, an oral cleft extending laterally, passing into the cheek, and extending to the lower eyelid with normal nasal alae is observed (Tessier cleft number 4). D-E: postoperative facial photographs at ten months old. Observe the asymmetry at the ocular region. F-K: computed tomography scans obtained at six months old. Note the right alveolar cleft extending laterally to the piriform aperture and finishing at the inner canthus (arrow) (Tessier cleft number 4). On the left side, a narrowing of the maxillozygomatic region leads to abnormal growth of zygomatic bone and a narrow temporozygomatic suture is observed (arrow in Figure H). Figure H also demonstrates the left lower orbital rim displaced upward compared to the right side. The left mandibular incisure is hypoplastic. Figure I is a CT axial section showing the right maxillary cleft and the left zygomatic cleft (Tessier number 7). Figure J reveals a right alveolar cleft until the infraorbital foramen in the inferior orbital rim (Tessier cleft number 4). Figure K demonstrates the hypoplastic zygomatic body with a cleft near the temporozygomatic suture (Tessier cleft number 7).

Case 37

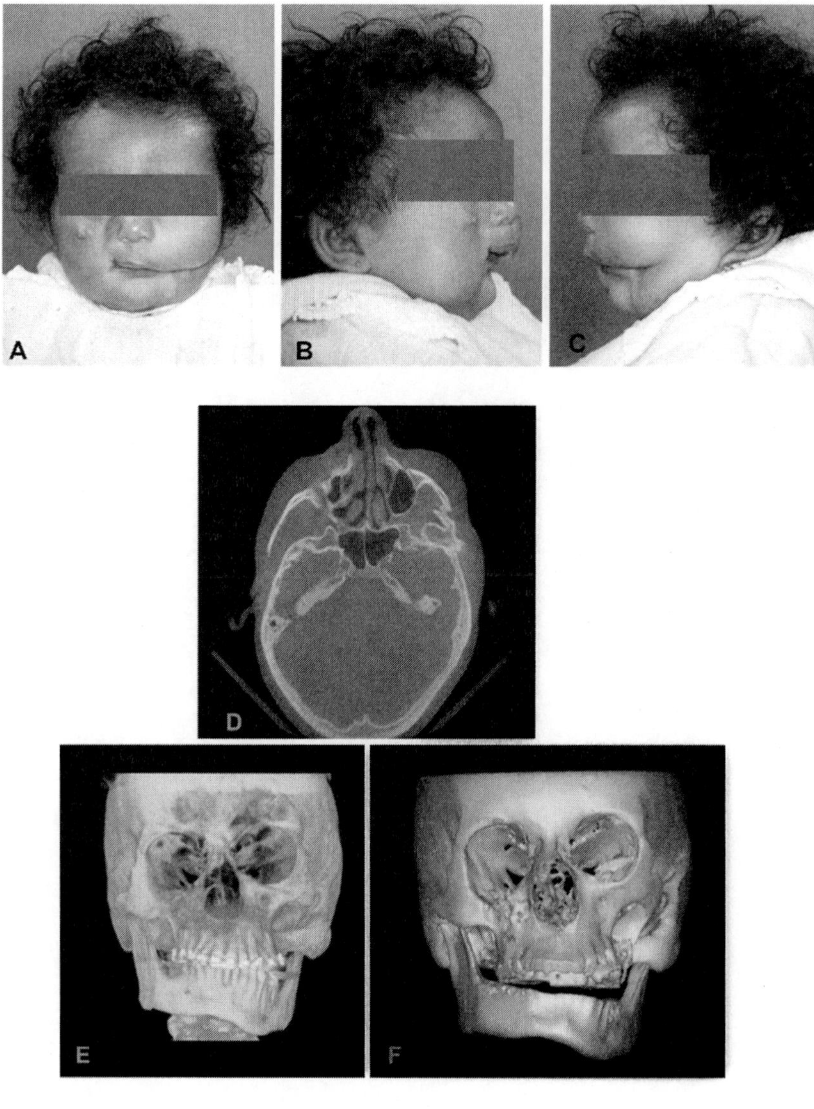

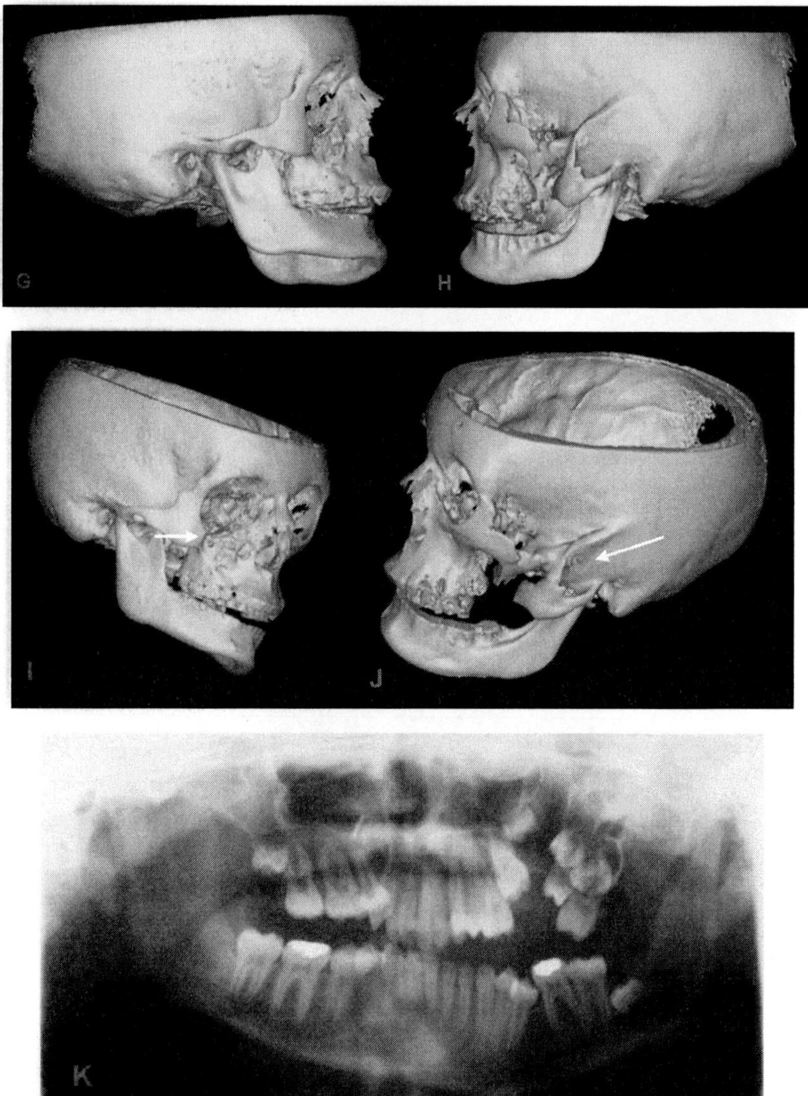
G
H
I
J
K

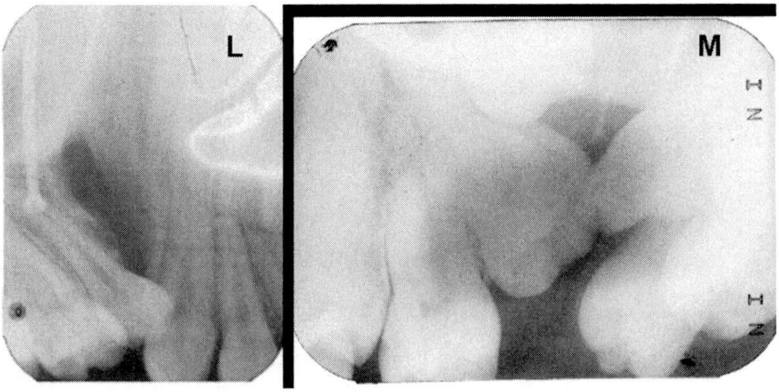

Figure 46 – Female patient with a left Tessier cleft number 7 on the left side. A-C: clinical phenotype of a female patient at seven months old with a Tessier cleft number 4 on the right side and number 7 on the left. Note the broad forehead, a sparse eyebrow, a short palpebral fissure, a short nose and the skin tags on the cheek on the right side. A small lateral notch in the upper lip vermilion on the right side extends to the ocular region as a notch (Tessier cleft number 4). Observe the left incomplete lateral cleft that extends from the macrostomia across the cheek towards the preauricular region (Tessier cleft number 7). D-J: computed tomography images performed at 19 years old. D: axial section showing the maxillary cleft on the right side and a fold in the zygomatic complex on the left side (arrows). E: frontal translucent image showing the asymmetry in both the midface and the mandible. F-H: CT 3D reconstructions revealing the frontal and lateral view orbital asymmetry, the midface hypoplasia, the oro-ocular cleft on the right side with a wide orbital floor cleft, an abnormal zygomatic arch on the left side and an asymmetric mandible. I-J: oblique views show a right cleft in the maxillary frontal process and inferior orbital rim (Tessier cleft number 4). Observe on the left side a severely malformed and displaced zygomatic complex with a fold segmenting the structure from the temporal bone (Tessier cleft number 7), an apparent duplication of the zygomatic arch and a disconnection between the zygomatic arches and the maxilla. On the left side, the maxillary region anchors in the upper region of the temporal bone (arrow). K-M: panoramic and periapical radiograph at 15 years old showing bilateral maxillary alveolar defect between the canine and first premolar (13–14) on the right and between the first and second premolar (24–25) on the left.

Case 38

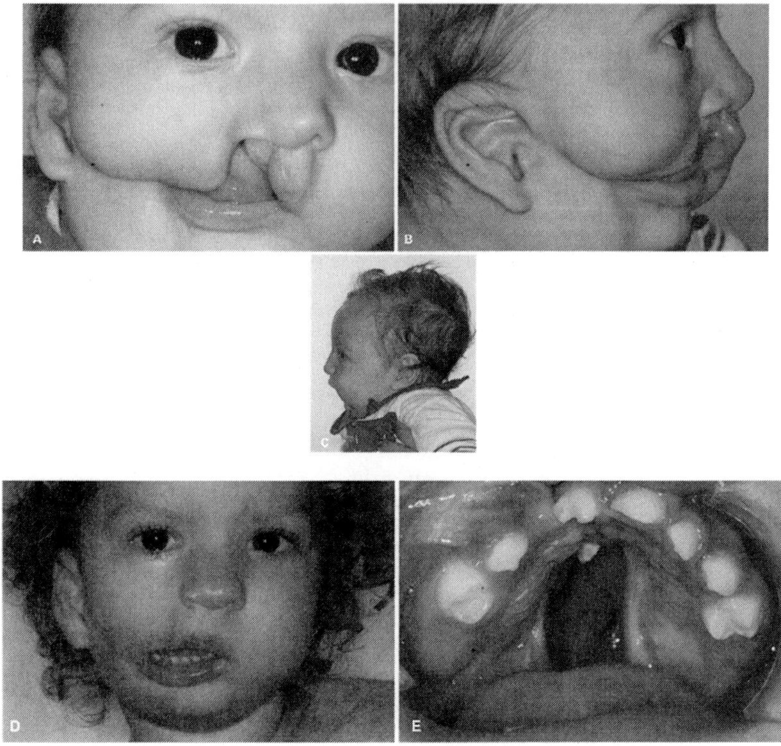

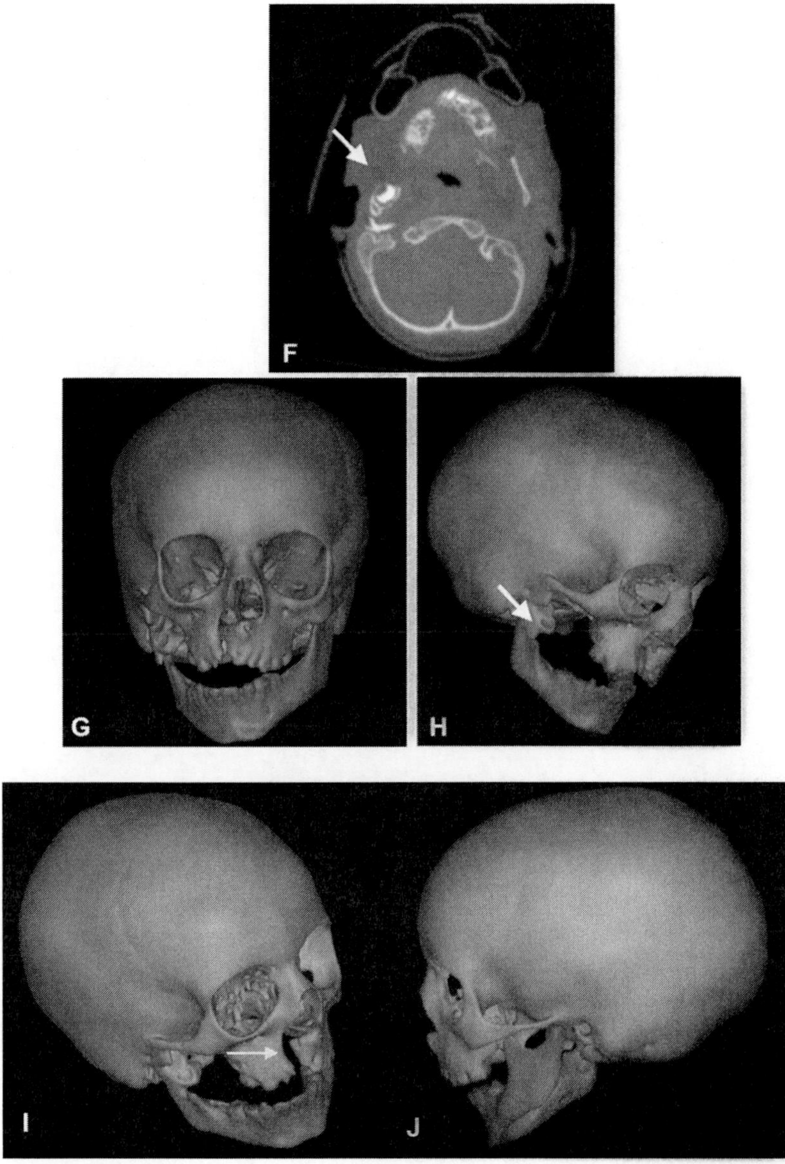

Figure 47 – Male patient with a right Tessier cleft number 7 associated with a right unilateral complete cleft lip and palate. A-C: clinical phenotype at three months old. Note a complete right lateral cleft running from the oral

commissure up to the tragus of the ear (Tessier cleft number 7) with macrostomia and the left side of the face without malformation. D: clinical phenotype at 2.8 years old showing the repaired clefts, an asymmetric face with a hypoplastic left mandibular ramus and a deviation of the right oral commissure. E: intraorally, a right unilateral complete cleft lip and palate was seen. F-J: computed tomography exam taken at three years old. Figure F is an axial section showing the right cleft in the alveolar arch and zygomatic bone (arrow). Figures G to J display a cleft in the alveolar arch (classical cleft) and a vertically hypoplastic maxillary. The right zygomatic body is hypoplastic, with the zygomatic arch displaced upwards. An additional bone structure downward outgrowth is seen in the temporal portion of the arch (arrow). The mandible is asymmetric, with a deformed right mandibular ramus and condyle. Agenesis of the coronoid process was also observed on the right side.

Although there is disagreement in the classification of some clefts in complex cases like this, we chose to classify this case as cleft number 7, according to Tessier (1976), because the cleft runs from the labial commissure to the tragus.

Published in: Pellerin, Philippe, Cristiano Tonello, Renato da Silva Freitas, Xiao Jun Tang, e Nivaldo Alonso. 2022. “Tessier’s Cleft Number 6 Revisited: A Series of 26 New Cases and Literature Review of 44”. *The Cleft Palate-Craniofacial Journal: Official Publication of the American Cleft Palate-Craniofacial Association*, 105566562210864. https://doi.org/10.1177/10556656221086459.

Case 39

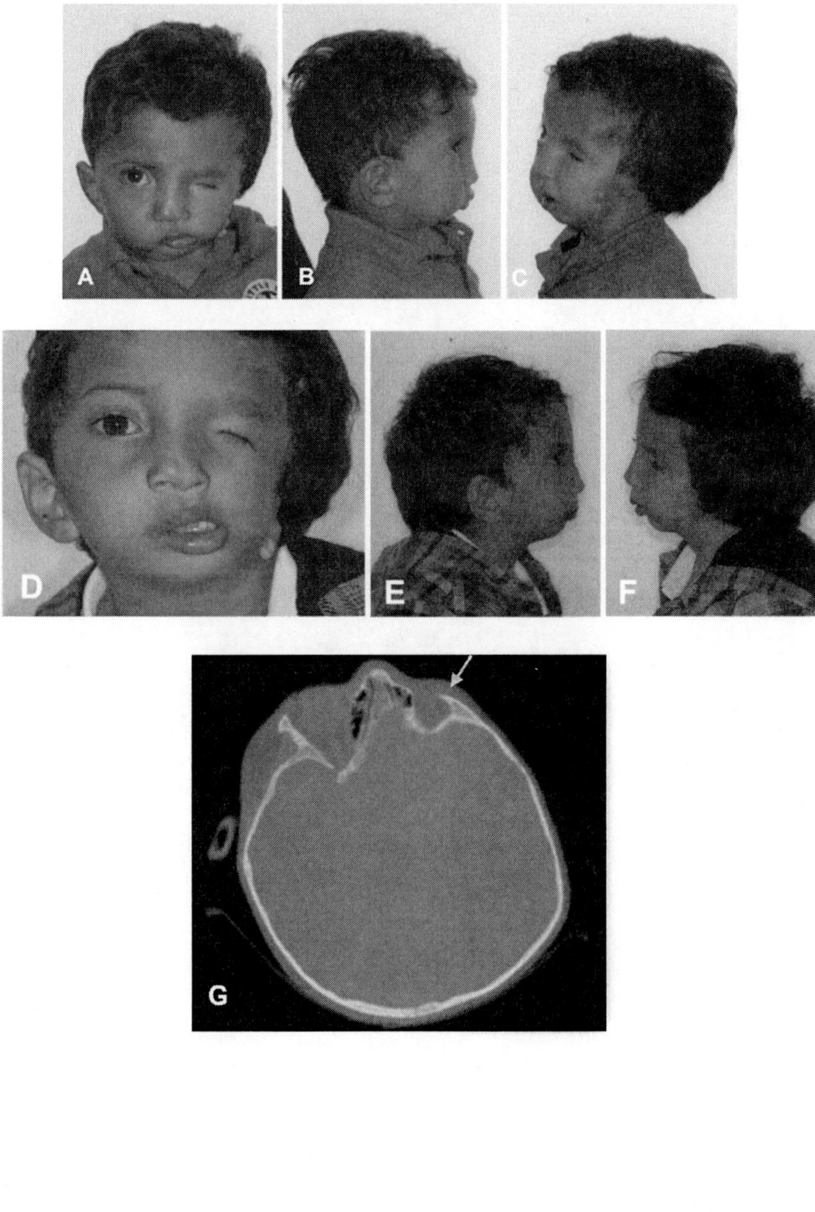

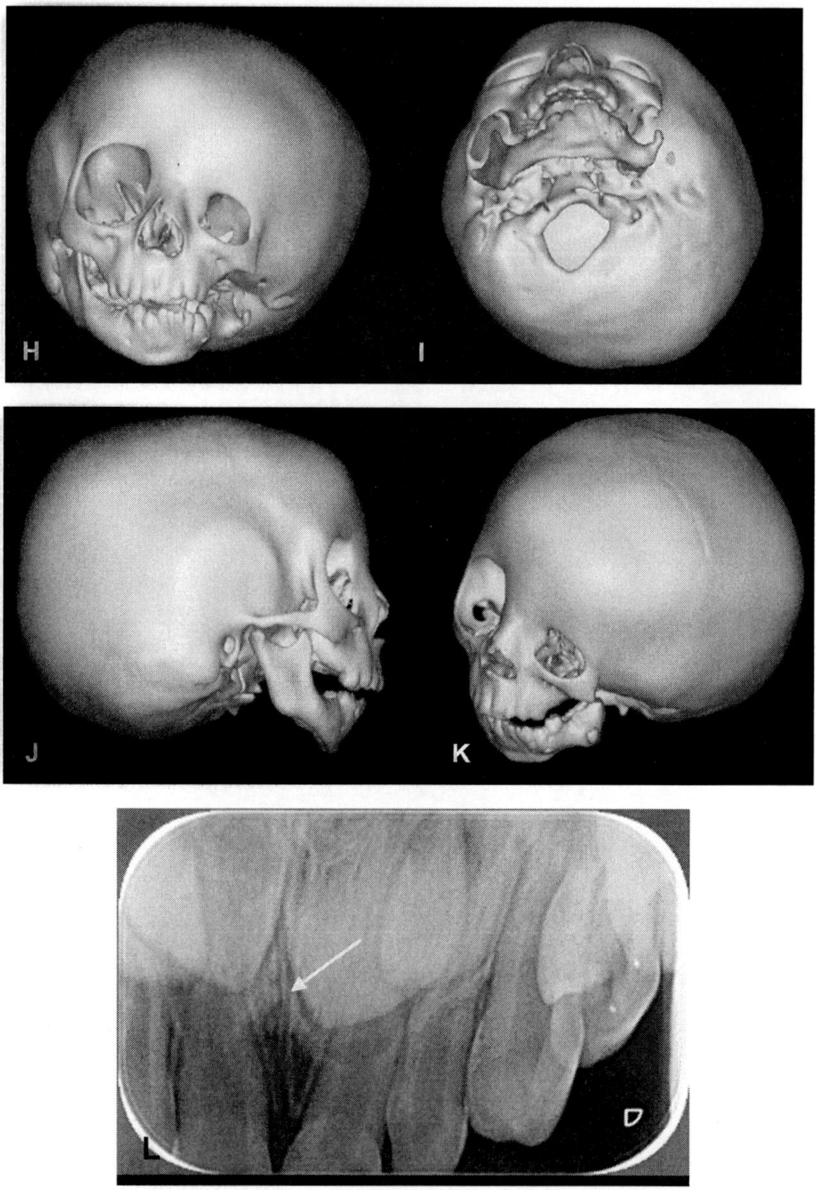

Figure 48 – Male patient with a left Tessier cleft number 7 associated with the oculoauriculovertebral spectrum. A-C: clinical phenotype at one and a

half years old. Note the facial asymmetry, the broad forehead, the microphthalmia, a slight bifid nasal tip, a microstomia, severe micrognathia and a left type III microtia with external auditory canal agenesis. D-F: revaluation of facial phenotype at three and a half years old. G-K: computed tomography exam obtained at nearly two years old. Figure G is an axial section at the level of the ocular cavity showing the left microphthalmia/anophthalmia. Figures H to K are CT 3D reconstructions demonstrating facial asymmetry, reduced left orbital size, and a complete absence of the left zygomatic arch (Tessier cleft number 7 or temporozygomatic cleft). A micrognathia associated with a mandibular anomaly with agenesis of the mandibular ramus, condyle, coronoid process, glenoid fossa and external meatus acoustic was observed on the left side. L: periapical radiography showing a slight midline defect of the alveolar region between the maxillary central incisors (Tessier cleft number 0).

CHAPTER NINE

TESSIER CLEFT NUMBER 8: THE FRONTOZYGOMATIC CLEFT

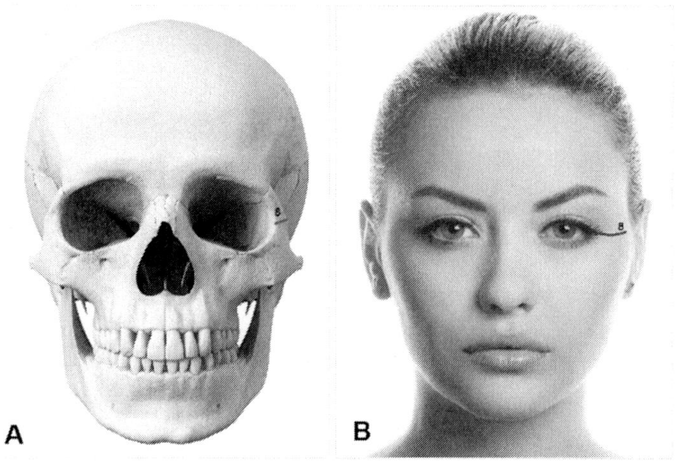

Figure 49 – Localization of Tessier cleft number 8. (A) Bone clefts numbered. (B) Soft tissue clefts numbered. Original artwork by the authors.

Tessier cleft number 8, also called the frontozygomatic cleft, is characterized by the absence of the lateral margin of the orbit in bone tissue and may be associated with an ocular globe anomaly (Figure 49). Anatomically, the soft tissue between the upper and lower eyelids is disrupted, and the continuity of the orbicularis muscle and the lateral bone is affected. Tessier cleft number 8 is frequently observed in cases with Treacher Collins syndrome, oculoauriculovertebral spectrum, amniotic band sequence and complex cases with multiple Tessier clefts.

References

David, D. J., M. H. Moore, and R. D. Cooter. 1989. "Tessier Clefts Revisited with a Third Dimension." *The Cleft Palate Journal* 26 (3): 163–84; discussion 184-5.

Lessa, Sergio, Roberto Sebastiá and Joao Pontello. 2019. "Lateral Canthal Clefts of the Eyelid." *Ophthalmic Plastic and Reconstructive Surgery* 35 (5): 491–94. https://doi.org/10.1097/iop.0000000000001353.

Tessier, Paul. 1976. "Anatomical Classification of Facial, Cranio-Facial and Latero-Facial Clefts." *Journal of Maxillofacial Surgery* 4: 69–92. https://doi.org/10.1016/s0301-0503(76)80013-6.

Winters, Ryan. 2016. "Tessier Clefts and Hypertelorism". *Facial Plastic Surgery Clinics of North America* 24 (4): 545–58. https://doi.org/10.1016/j.fsc.2016.06.013.

Tessier cleft number 8

Case 40

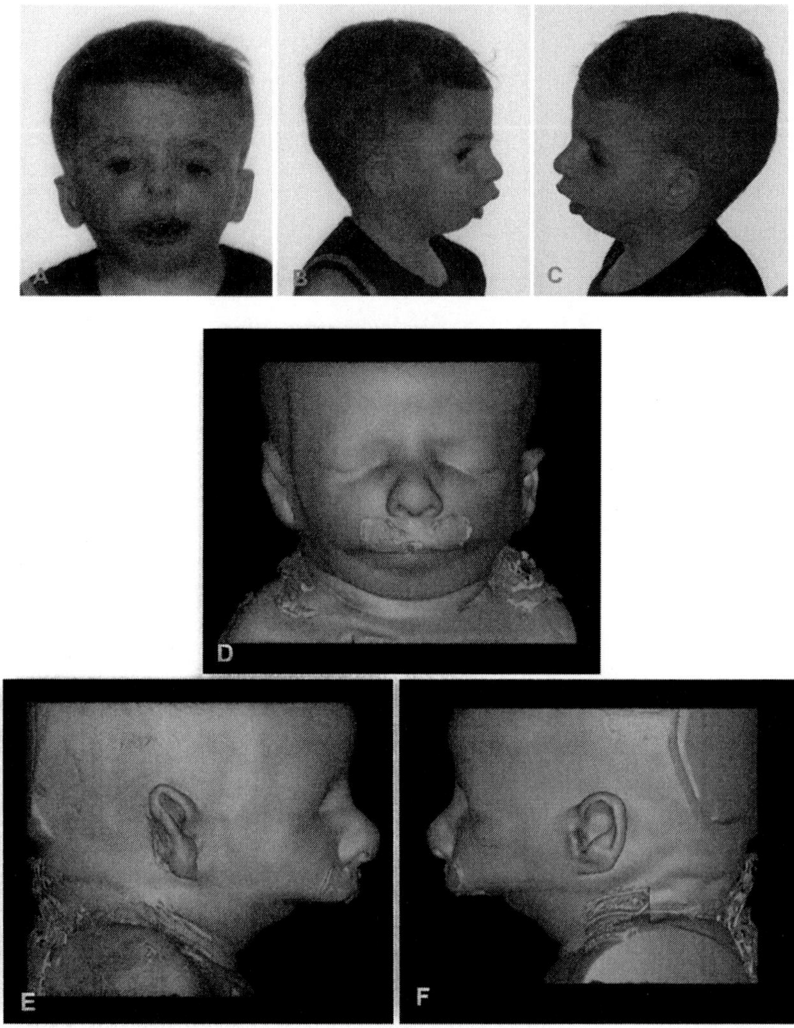

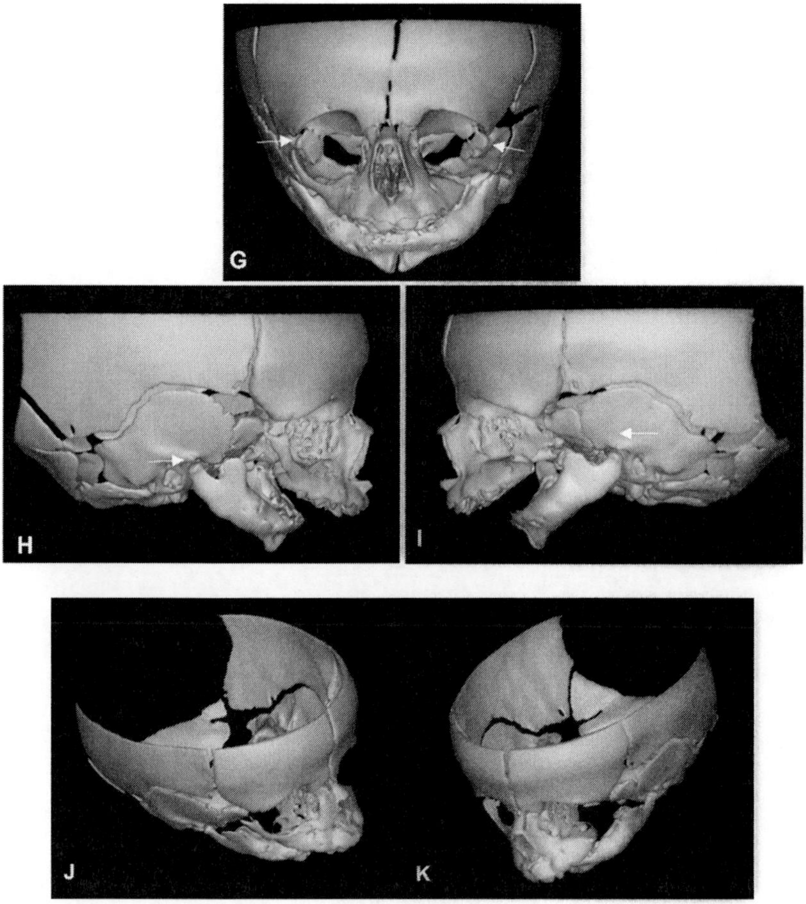

Figure 50 – Male patient with a Tessier cleft number 8 on the right side associated with Nager syndrome. A-C: clinical phenotype at two years old. Note in the soft tissue the broad forehead, the down slanting palpebral fissure, the extremely severe micrognathia and the abnormal ears. D-K: computed tomography images taken at 19 days old. Figures D-F show the soft tissue reconstruction demonstrating the down-slanting palpebral fissure and micrognathia. Figures G to K reveal the hard tissue with a bilateral frontozygomatic cleft (Tessier cleft number 8) associated with a bilateral hypoplasia of the zygomatic bone. On the left side, a hypoplastic lateral orbital rim on the right side and a complete absence of the lateral (arrow) and infraorbital rim (maxillary-zygomatic cleft—Tessier number 6).

Figures H to I display bilateral agenesis of the zygomatic arch (Tessier cleft number 7—temporozygomatic cleft—arrow) and severe micrognathia. Figures J and K show an oblique view of the Tessier cleft number 8. Due to the early age of the patient in the CT exam, the cranial sutures and the midline mandible synchondrosis were not closed.

Case 41

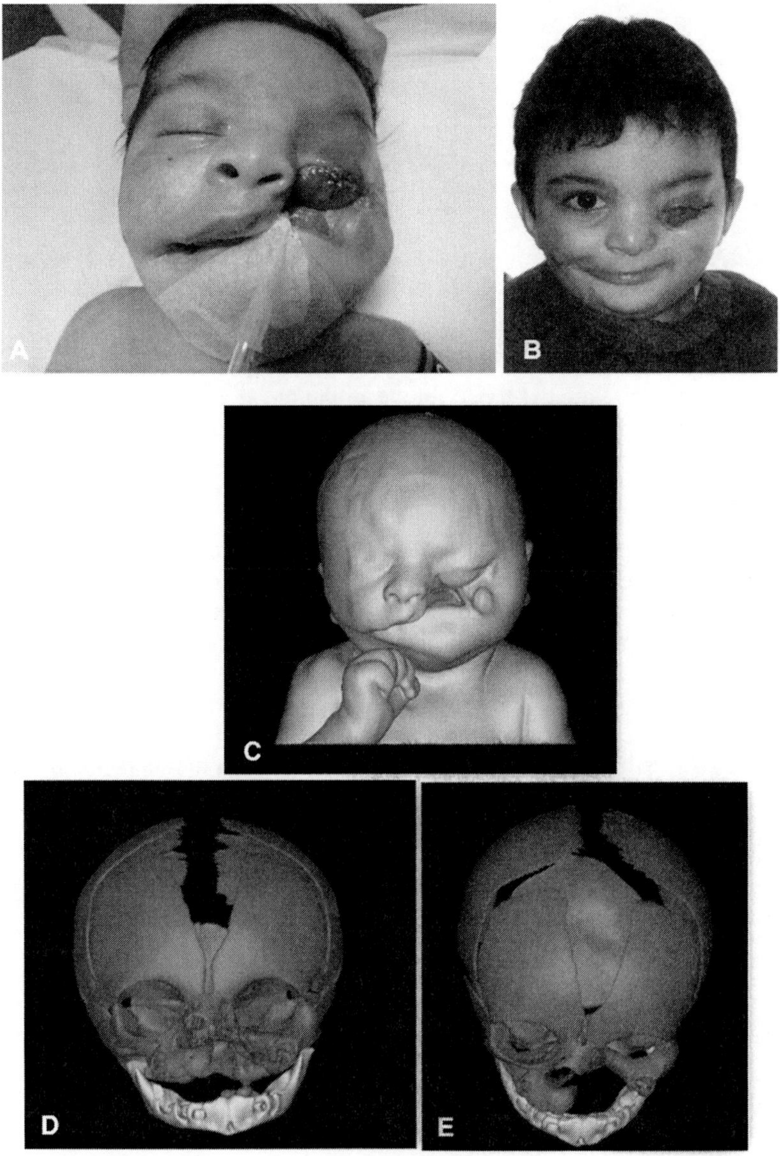

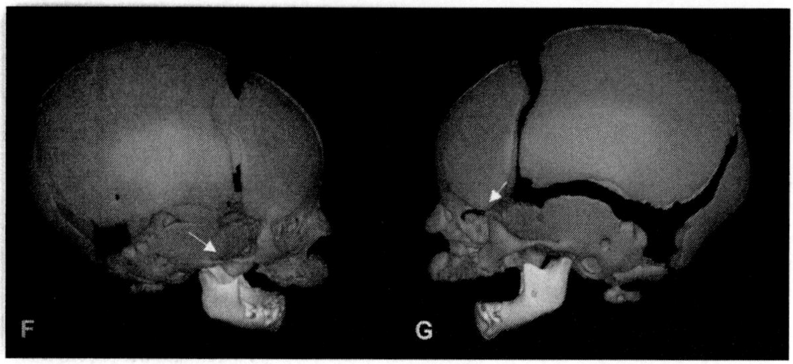

Figure 51 – Male patient with a Tessier cleft number 8 on the left side associated with the amniotic band sequence. (A) the clinical phenotype at one month old. Note the broad forehead, the facial and orbital asymmetry, an extremely wide left cleft lip, and palate extending to the ocular inner canthus (Tessier cleft number 4 or orbito-maxillary cleft) and laterally to the infraorbital foramen and the ocular outer canthus with direct communication between the orbit, maxillary bone and oral cavity at left. An upper eyelid hypoplastic with absent eyelashes and severe exposure of the ocular globe was present. On the right side, note the lateral cleft with macrostomia (Tessier cleft number 7). B: clinical phenotype at age one and half years, showing the repaired clefts. C-G: computed tomography 3D images obtained on the day of birth. In Figure C, note the soft tissue complex association of Tessier clefts. Figures D to E demonstrate the hard tissue 3D reconstruction revealing a left wide orbito-maxillary cleft with agenesis of the maxillary bone and infraorbital rim (Tessier cleft numbers 4 and 5). In Figure F, note a slight zygomatic arch cleft on the right side (arrow—Tessier cleft number 7). Figure G shows a left cleft in the lateral orbital rim (arrow—Tessier cleft number 8).

CHAPTER TEN

TESSIER CLEFT NUMBER 9: THE SUPEROLATERAL ORBITAL CLEFT

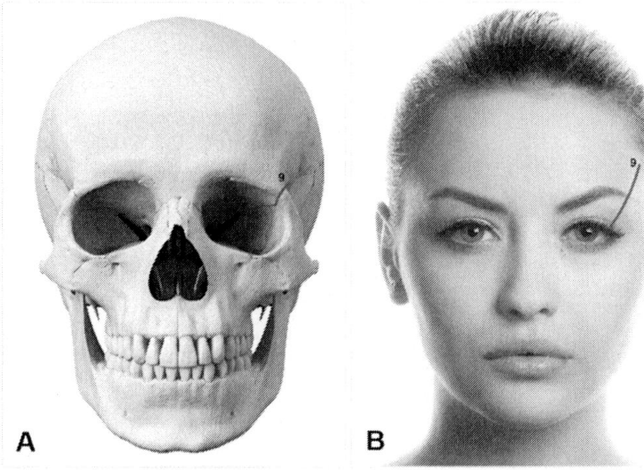

Figure 52 – Localization of Tessier cleft number 9. (A) Bone clefts numbered. (B) Soft tissue clefts numbered. Original artwork by the authors.

Tessier cleft number 9 is a rare superolateral orbital cleft that extends to the temporal fossa. In the soft tissue, a groove in the orbicularis muscle of the eye may be present, and the superolateral rim and wall may be absent. In bone tissue, it is characterized as a bone cleft, or notch, affecting the upper portion of the orbit and the temporal fossa (adjacent to the parietal bone) (Figure 52).

References

Bubanale, Shivanand Chanabasu, Santosh B. Kurbet, and Linda Maria Genoveva De Piedade Sequeira. 2017. "A Rare Case of Cleft Number Nine Associated with Atypical Cleft Number Two." *Indian Journal of Ophthalmology* 65 (7): 610–12. https://doi.org/10.4103/ijo.IJO_914_16.

David, D. J., M. H. Moore, and R. D. Cooter. 1989. "Tessier Clefts Revisited with a Third Dimension." *The Cleft Palate Journal* 26 (3): 163–84; discussion 184-5.

David, David J., Mark H. Moore, Rodney D. Cooter, and Sik-Kuen Chow. 1989. "The Tessier Number 9 Cleft." *Plastic and Reconstructive Surgery* 83 (3): 520–25. https://doi.org/10.1097/00006534-198903000-00022.

Pereira, Filipe J., Gherusa H. Milbratz, Antonio A. V. Cruz, and João J. A. Vasconcelos. 2010. "Ophthalmic Considerations in the Management of Tessier Cleft 5/9." Ophthalmic Plastic and Reconstructive Surgery 26 (6): 450–53. https://doi.org/10.1097/IOP.0b013e3181d9293a.

Tessier, Paul. 1976. "Anatomical Classification of Facial, Cranio-Facial and Latero-Facial Clefts." *Journal of Maxillofacial Surgery* 4: 69–92. https://doi.org/10.1016/s0301-0503(76)80013-6.

Winters, Ryan. 2016. "Tessier Clefts and Hypertelorism". *Facial Plastic Surgery Clinics of North America* 24 (4): 545–58. https://doi.org/10.1016/j.fsc.2016.06.013.

Tessier cleft number 9

Case 42

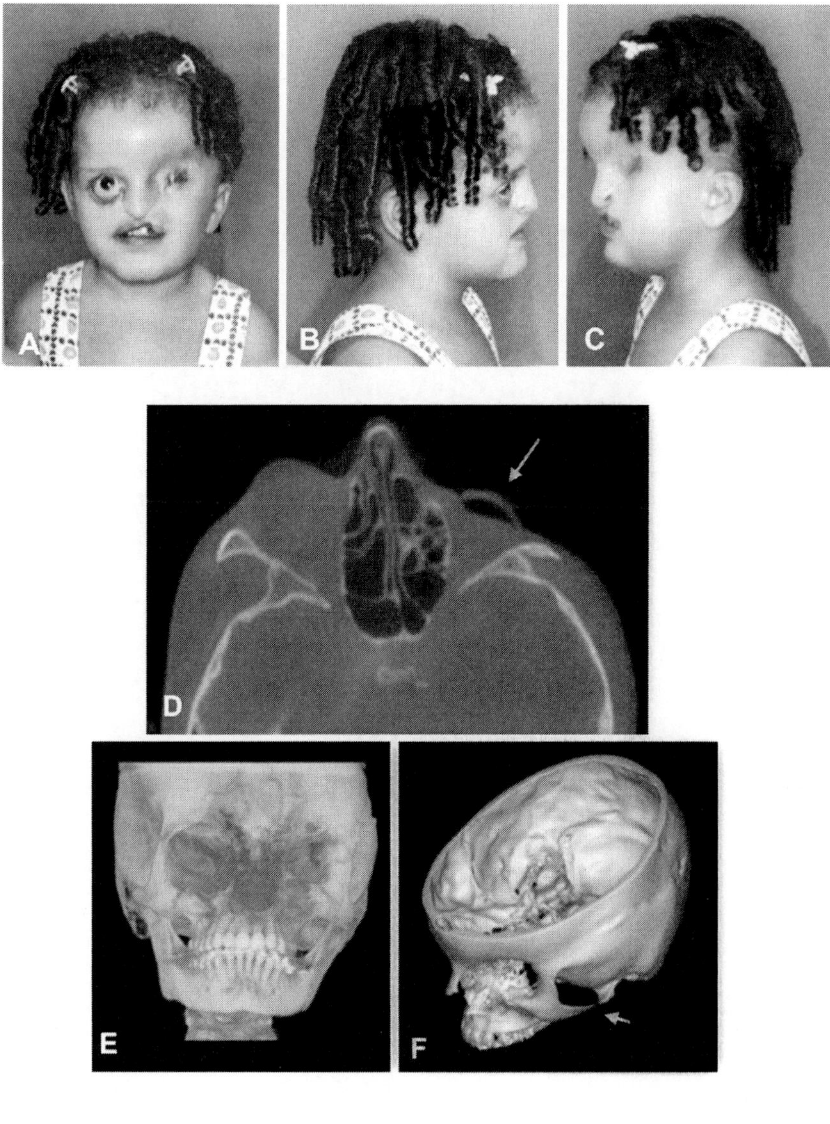

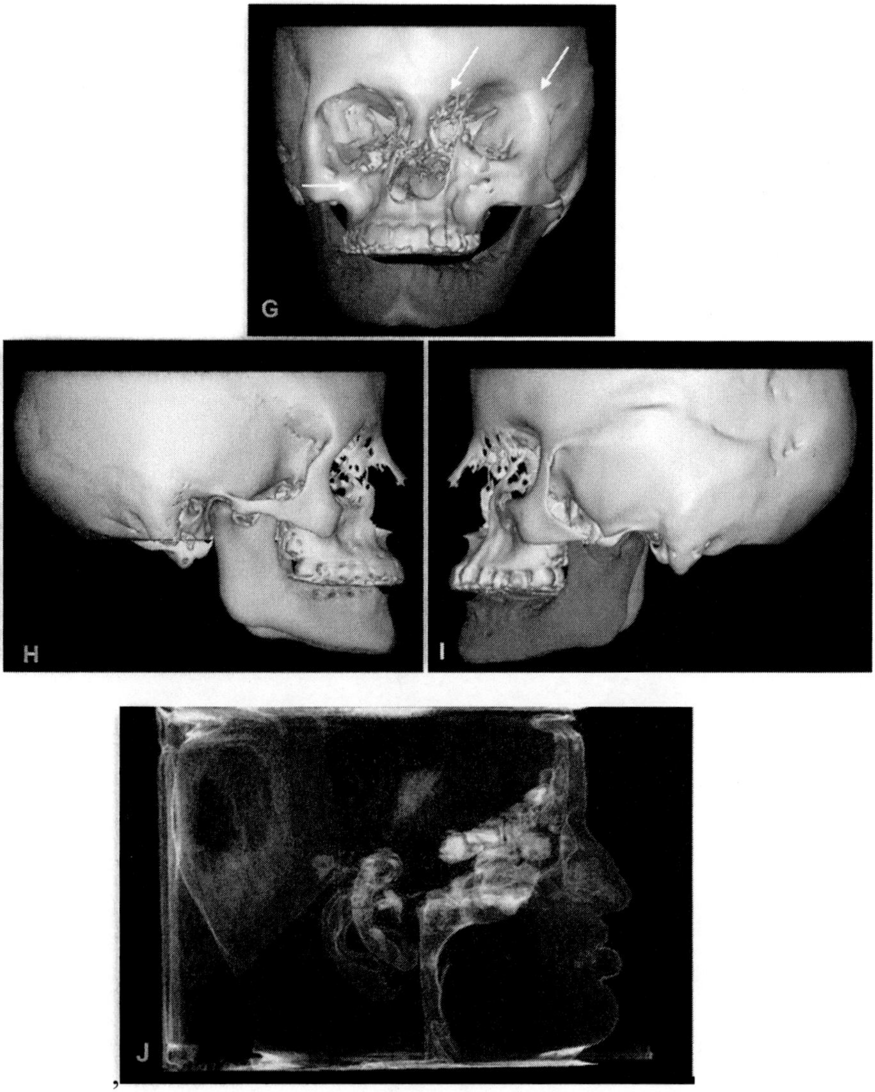
G
H
I
J

,

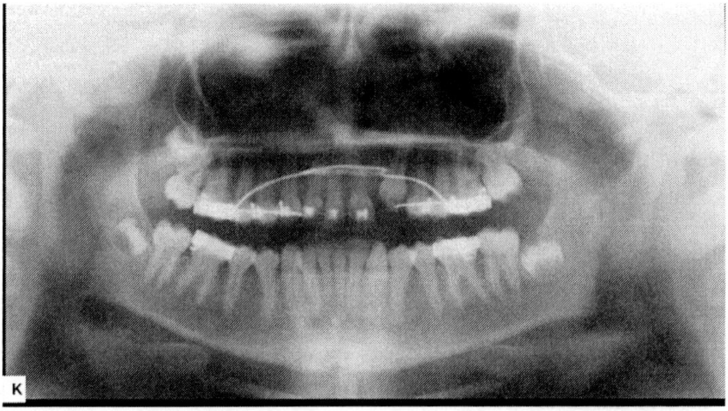

Figure 53– Female patient with a left Tessier cleft number 9. A-C: clinical phenotype at age five. Note the soft tissue in a broad forehead, facial asymmetry, a sparse bilateral eyebrow, a lower eyelid augmentation on the right side, left anophthalmia and deformity that extends from the lateral third of the upper eyelid through the lateral end of the eyebrow to the temporal scalp alopecia (Tessier cleft number 9). A midface hypoplasia, narrow nostrils with bilateral underdeveloped ala nasi, a left cleft lip and alveolus, a complete left, and an incomplete right oro-nasal-ocular cleft (Tessier cleft number 3) are seen. D-J: computed tomography exam taken at 16 years old. Figure D shows a CT axial section showing anophthalmia on the left side (arrow). Figure E is a translucent 3D reconstruction showing preserved bony structure in the maxilla and mandible. Figures F and I reveal a left deficient zygomatic arch with a temporozygomatic cleft (Tessier cleft number 7, arrow in Figure F) and a decreased orbital size on the left side. The nasal cavity is preserved, and the left bony failure in the nasal bone suggests Tessier cleft number 13, associated with a left superolateral orbital cleft extending to the temporal fossa (Tessier number 9). On the right side, an infraorbital rim hypoplastic suggests Tessier cleft number 6. J: an adequate upper airway is observed in a lateral view. (K) panoramic radiograph at 12 years old showing the absence of dental anomalies.

Case 43

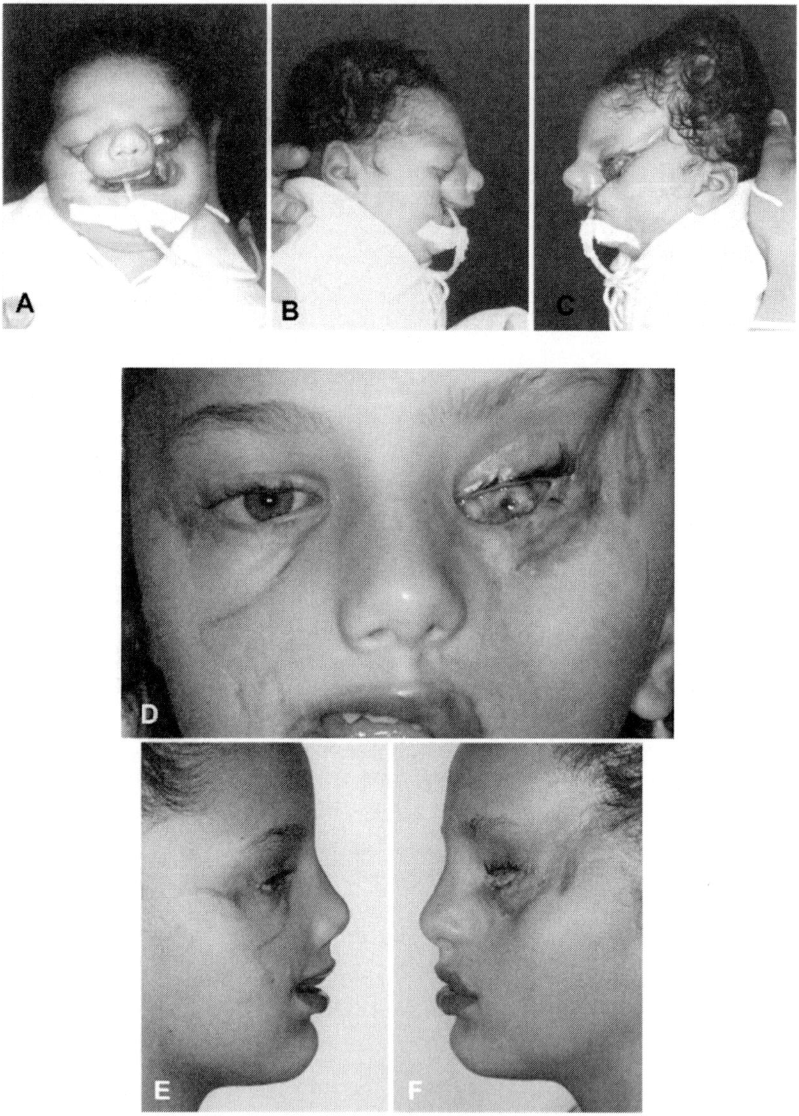

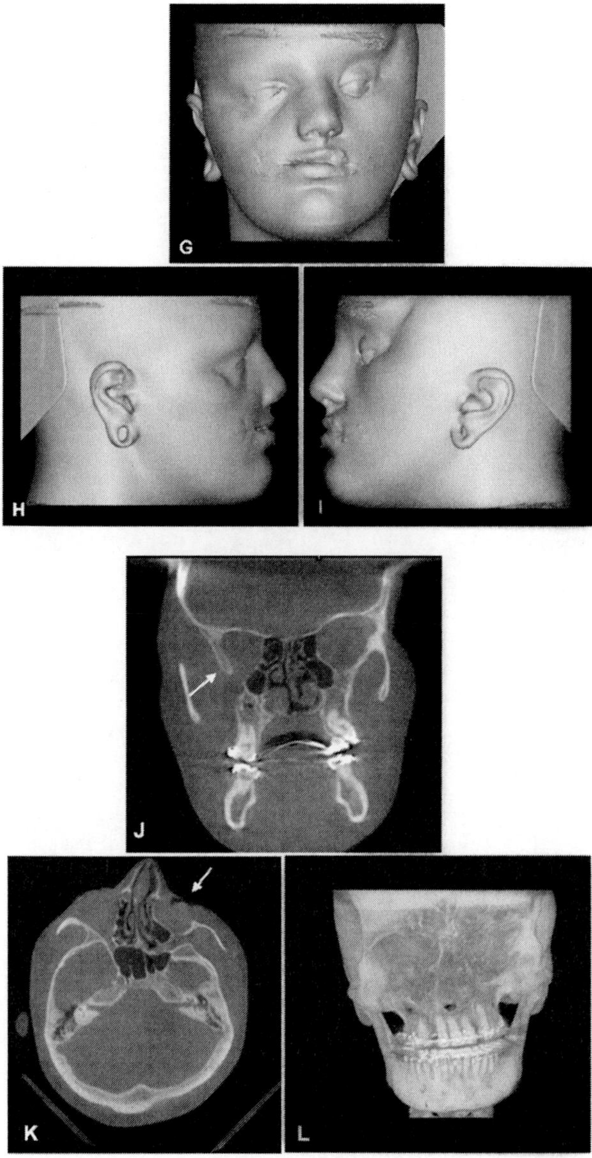
G
H
I
J
K
L

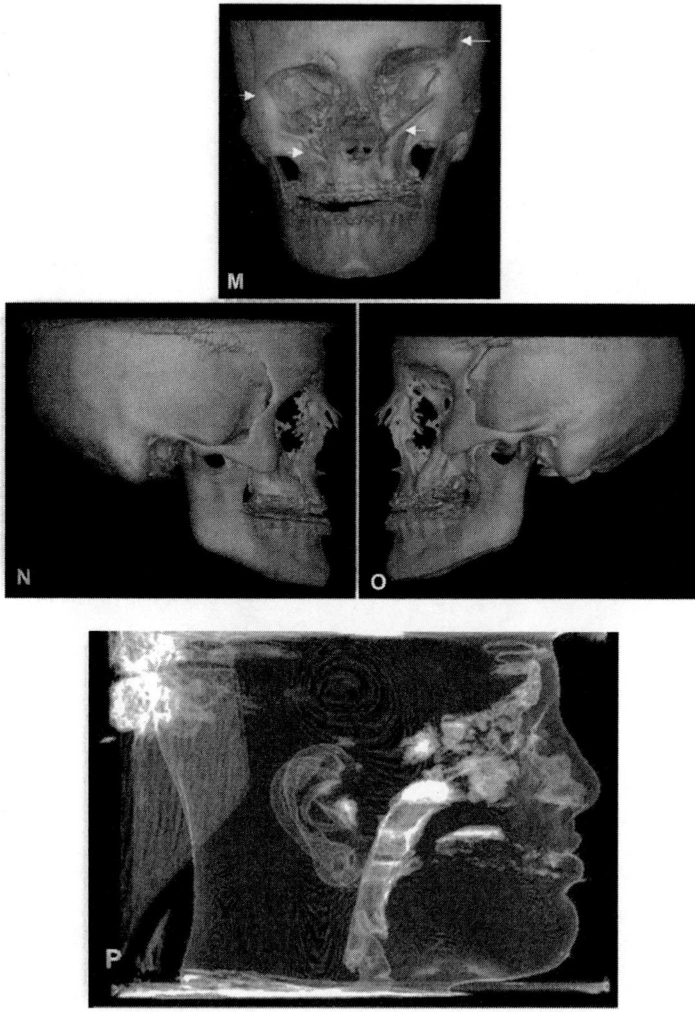
M
N
O
P

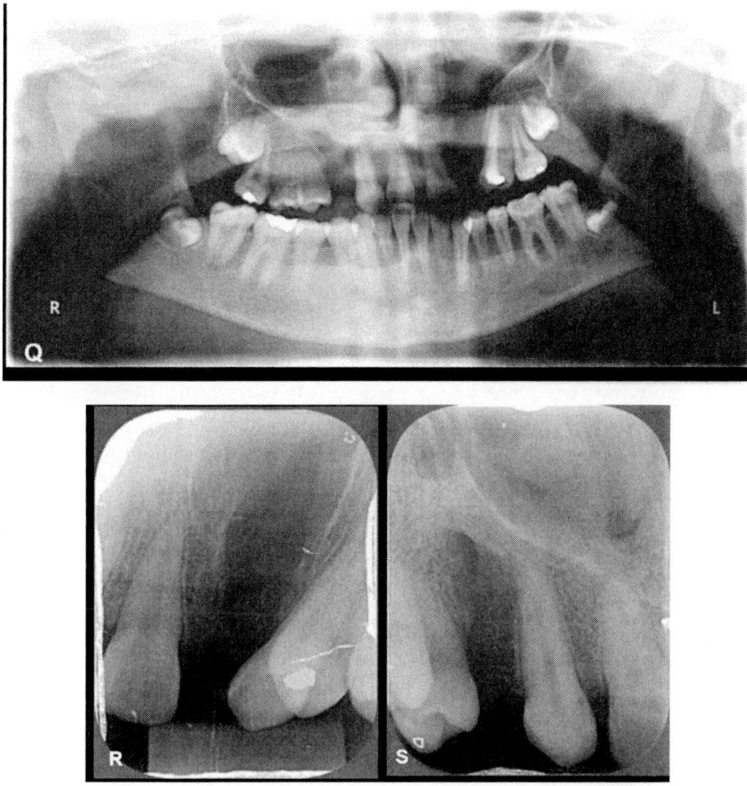

Figure 54 – Female patient with a left Tessier cleft number 9 with amniotic band sequence diagnosis (with complex craniofacial cleft and ring constriction). A-C: clinical phenotype at four months old. Note the premolar region's right cleft lip and alveolus extending superiorly until the infraorbital rim (Tessier cleft number 5). On the left side, note an orbito-maxillary cleft that starts in the upper lip and extends onto the cheek to the infraorbital eyelid (Tessier cleft number 4). The left cleft also extends to the lateral third of the upper eyelid affecting the supra-lateral orbital angle and the temporal fossa (Tessier cleft number 9). On the left side is a macrostomia with a mild medial-lateral cleft (Tessier cleft number 7). D-F: clinical phenotype at nine years old showing a short nose and repaired clefts. G-P: computed tomography images obtained at 17 years old. Soft tissue 3D reconstructions (Figures G to I) show a left-side deformity that extends from the lateral third of the upper eyelid through the lateral end of the eyebrow to the temporal bone (Tessier cleft number 9). Figures H and I demonstrate hypoplasia of

the lateral orbital rim on the right side, suggesting Tessier cleft number 8. Figure J is the CT coronal section showing the decreased orbital cavity on the left side. Figure K is an axial section showing microphthalmia (arrow). Figure L is a translucent 3D reconstruction showing a midface asymmetry and radiopaque orthodontic appliances. Figures M to O are CT 3D reconstructions of the hard tissue. On the right side is a dysplastic frontozygomatic bony with an abnormal lateral orbital rim (Tessier cleft number 8) and a bone cleft extending from the inferior orbital rim to the premolar region (Tessier cleft number 5). On the left side, note the superolateral orbital cleft extending to the temporal fossa (Tessier cleft number 9) and an orbito-maxillary-oral cleft that involves the maxillary inferior orbital rim and floor (Tessier cleft number 4). (P) the CT lateral view demonstrates a wide upper airway. Q: panoramic radiograph at 11 years old showing a bilateral alveolar defect between the canine and first premolar (13–14) on the right and central incisor and canine (21–23) on the left. R-S: periapical radiograph at 11 years old showing agenesis of the maxillary lateral incisors (12–22) bilaterally.

CHAPTER ELEVEN

TESSIER CLEFT NUMBER 10: THE LATERAL ORBITOFRONTAL EYELID AND ORBITAL RIM CLEFT

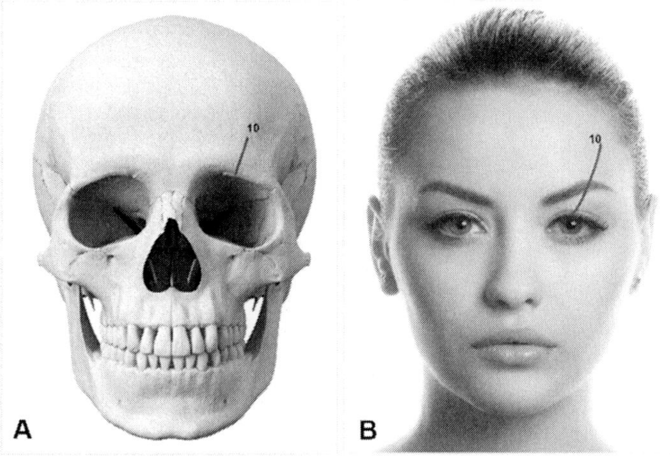

Figure 55 –Localization of Tessier cleft number 10. (A) Bone clefts numbered. (B) Soft tissue clefts numbered. Original artwork by the authors.

Tessier cleft number 10, or cleft of the lateral orbitofrontal region of the orbital rim, affects the middle third of the upper limit of the orbital cavity extending to the frontal bone with encephalocele and coloboma of the middle third of the upper eyelid. The eyebrow is divided into two portions, and the scalp is practically absent in the affected region; Figure 55.

References

Barnett JM, Pang JHY, Herman S, et al. Craniofacial Cleft: A Case of Tessier 10 Cleft with a Novel Method to Repair Large Bilateral Colobomas. *Cleft Palate Craniofac J.* 2019;56(10):1377-1380.

David DJ, Moore MH, Cooter RD. Tessier clefts revisited with a third dimension. *Cleft Palate J.* 1989;26(3):163–184, discussion 184–185.

David, David J., Mark H. Moore, Rodney D. Cooter, and Sik-Kuen Chow. 1989. "The Tessier Number 9 Cleft." *Plastic and Reconstructive Surgery* 83 (3): 520–25. https://doi.org/10.1097/00006534-198903000-00022.

Fan X, Shao C, Fu Y, Zhou H, Lin M, Zhu H. Surgical management and outcome of Tessier number 10 clefts. *Ophthalmology*. 2008; 115(12): 2290-2294.e3.

Shao C, Lu W, Li J, et al. Manifestation and grading of ocular involvement in patients with Tessier number 10 clefts. *Eye (Lond).* 2017;31(8):1140-1145.

Tessier, Paul. 1976. "Anatomical Classification of Facial, Cranio-Facial and Latero-Facial Clefts." *Journal of Maxillofacial Surgery* 4: 69–92.

Tessier cleft number 10

Case 44

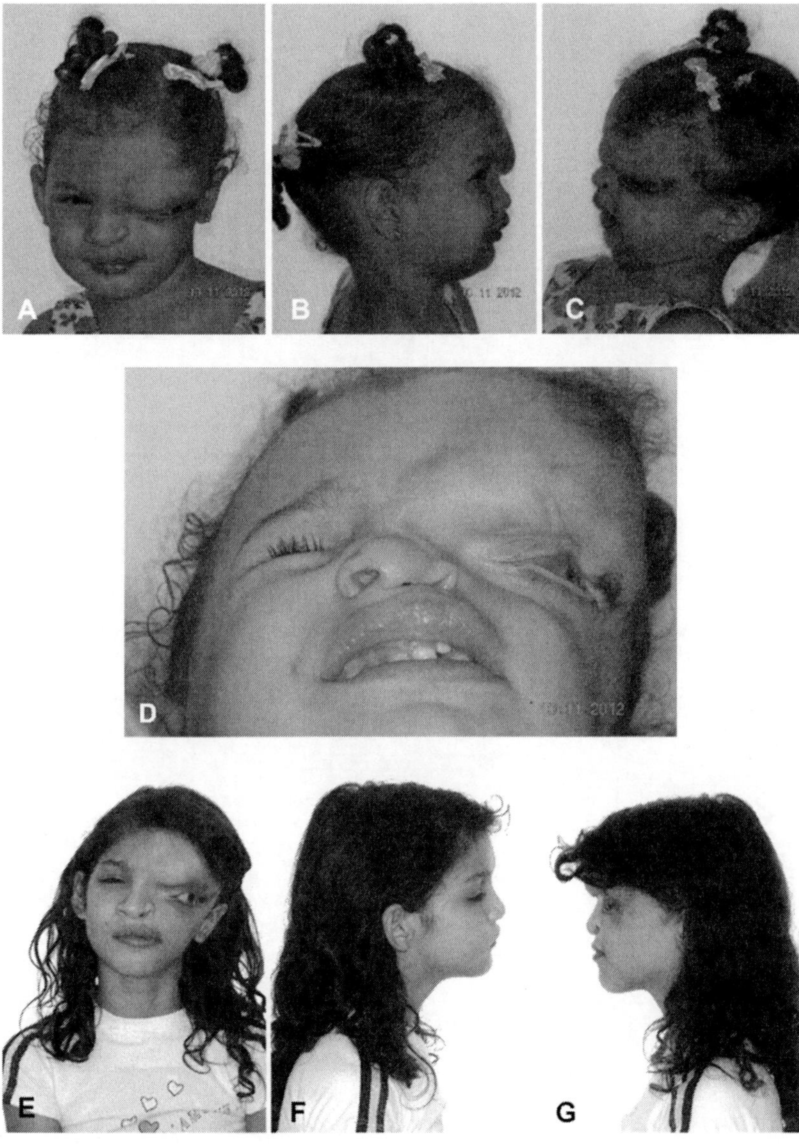

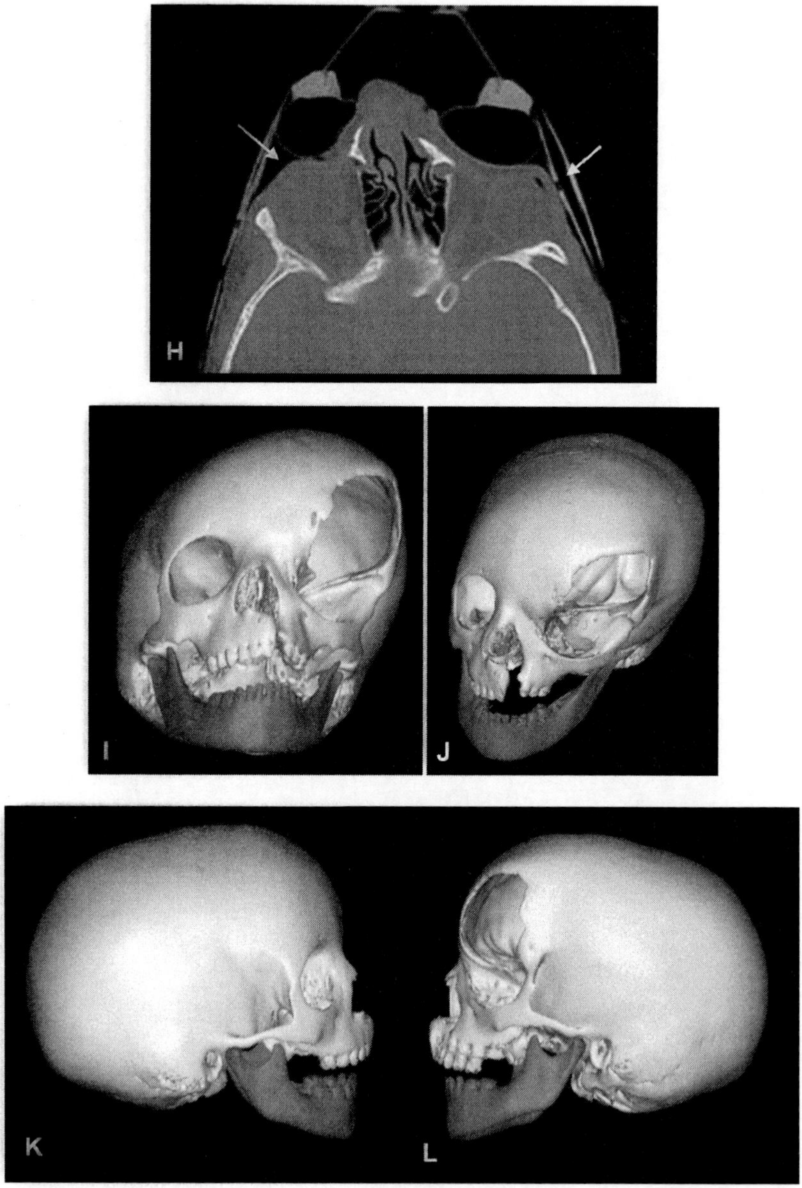
H
I
J
K
L

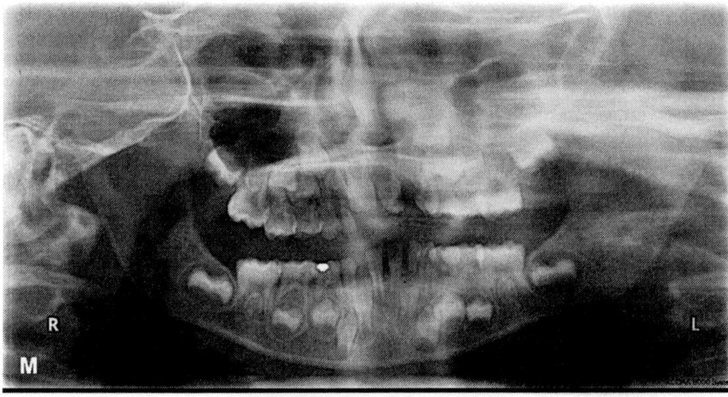

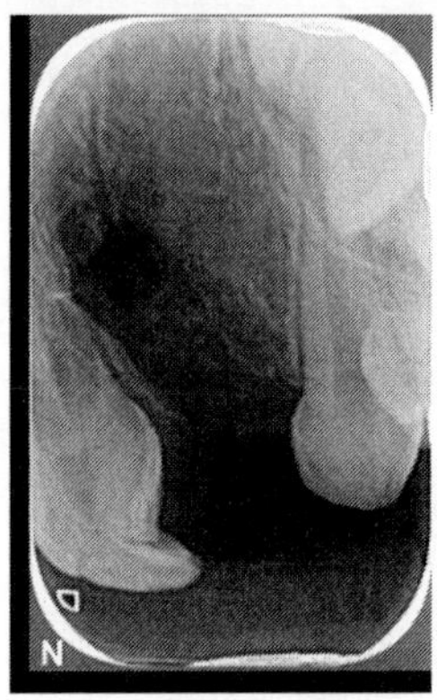

Figure 56– Female patient with a left Tessier cleft number 10. A-D: clinical phenotype at two years old. Note the broad forehead and the left supraorbital encephalocele. Ocular hypertelorism in the left hemiface, a severe facial asymmetry, an elongated palpebral fissure, absent eyebrows and a wide coloboma in the middle one-third of the upper eyelid (Tessier cleft number 10) are observed. A left cleft lip extends to the nasal region, displacing the alae nasi. This cleft continues to the maxillary region until the inner canthus of the eye (Tessier cleft number 3). Figure D shows a magnification of the frontal bony cleft with a left broad encephalocele and a cleft in the middle one-third of the upper eyelid. E-G: clinical phenotype at eight years old showing repaired clefts. H-L: computed tomography images obtained at five years old. Figure H is a CT axial section showing normal ocular globes (arrows). Figures I to L are CT 3D reconstructions. Note the left cleft in the alveolar arch extending to the nasal bone. The maxillozygomatic region is abnormal, with an irregular orbital rim. A wide left frontal bony cleft with

a large encephalocele involving the anterior half of the orbital roof, the supraorbital rim of the frontal bone (Tessier cleft number 10) is seen. A left cleft of the superolateral margin of the orbit (Tessier cleft number 9) is also observed. M-N: panoramic and periapical radiograph at seven years old showing agenesis of the maxillary lateral incisor (22) at left and maxillary alveolar defect.

Case 45

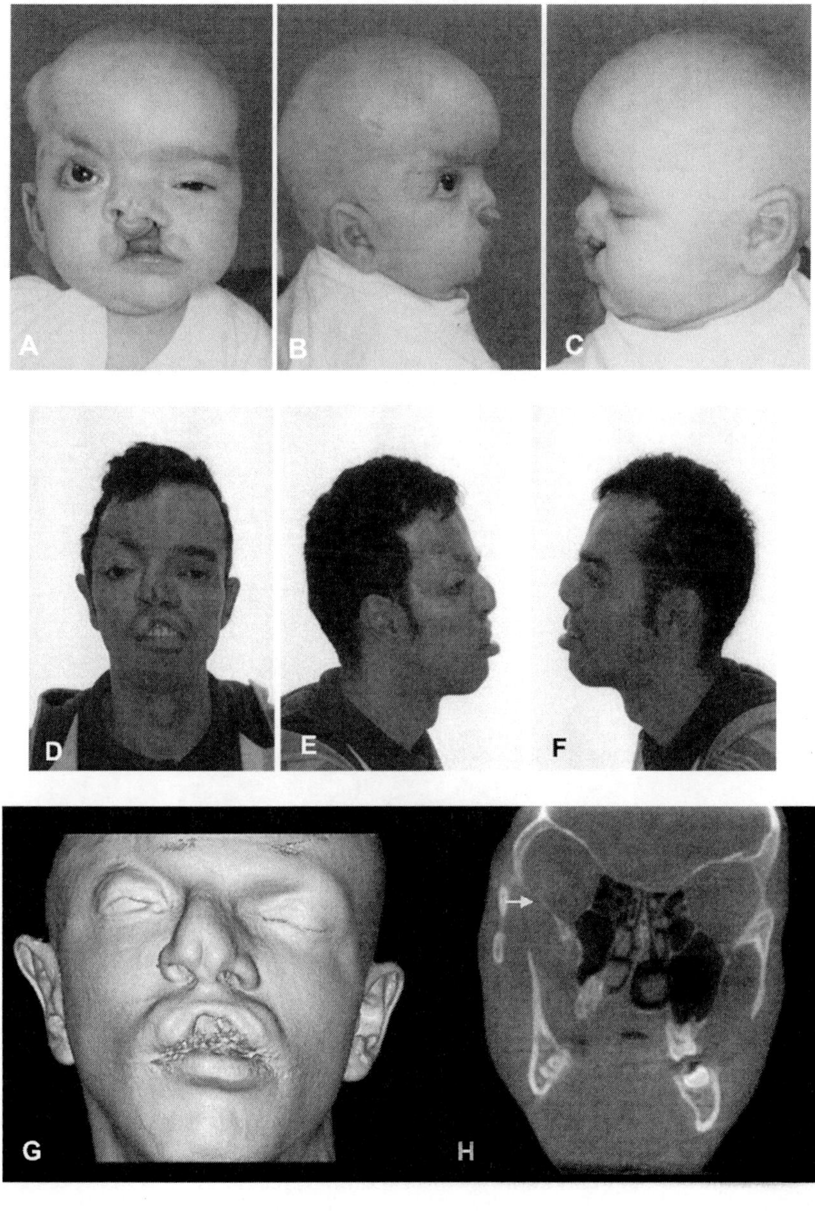

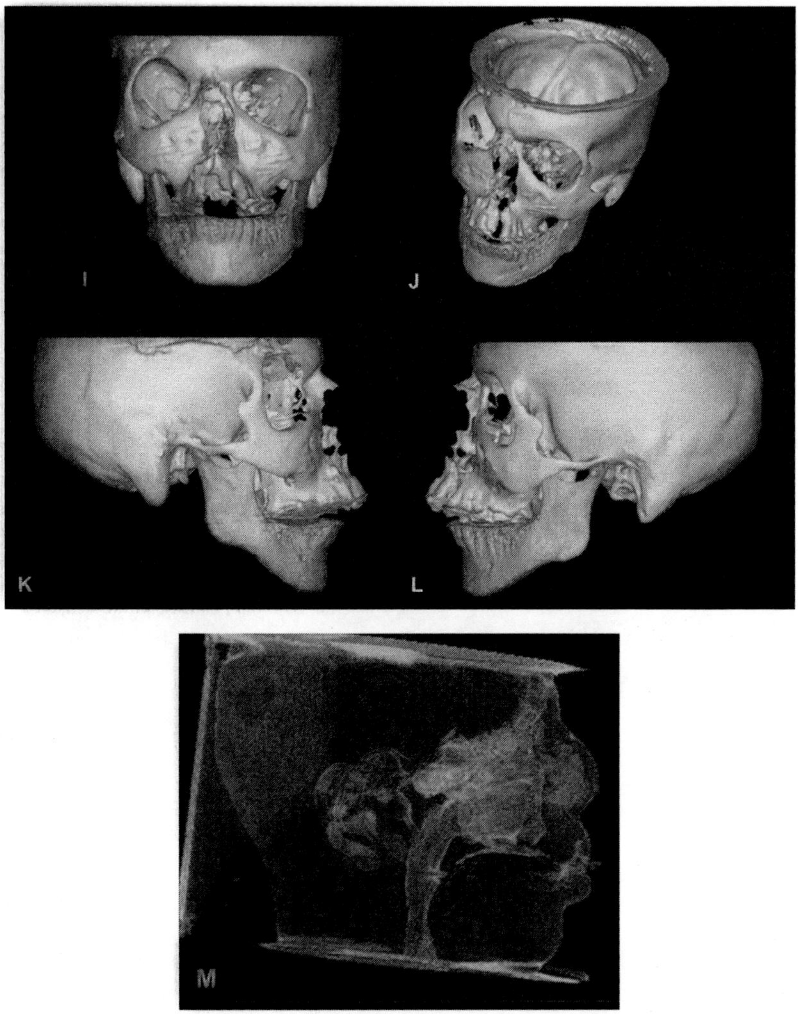

Figure 57 – Male patient with a right Tessier cleft number 10 with amniotic bands sequence. A-E: clinical phenotype at two months old. Note the right frontal bossing and the coloboma of the medial upper eyelid (Tessier cleft number 10) associated with a parietal bone encephalocele on the right side. Ocular hypertelorism, facial asymmetry, a depressed nasal bridge, and a slight nasal tip bifidity (Tessier cleft number 0) were observed. A bilateral complete cleft lip and palate with protruding premaxilla was also present. D-F: clinical phenotype at 29 years old showing an elongated face and

repaired clefts. G-L: computed tomography exam obtained at 29 years old. Note in the soft tissue (Figure G) a discontinuous supraorbital bridge (Tessier cleft number 10), a nasal tip bifidity (Tessier number 0) and a short philtrum as an outcome of cleft lip repair. Figure H is a CT coronal section showing the orbit asymmetry and the nasal septum deviation. Figures I to L are CT 3D reconstructions of the hard tissue. Note the wide and asymmetric orbital cavity with bone failure on the right side (arrow in Figure J), the frontal bossing, the protruded premaxilla and the left alveolar cleft. (M) airway view.

CHAPTER TWELVE

TESSIER CLEFT NUMBER 11: THE SUPEROMEDIAL EYELID AND ORBITAL RIM CLEFT

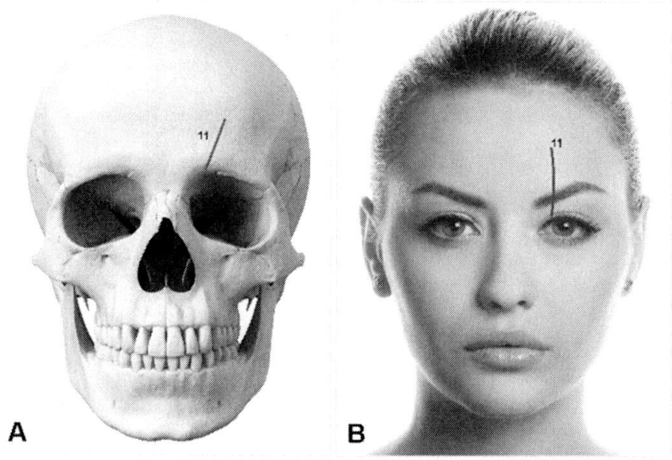

Figure 58 –Localization of Tessier cleft number 11. (A) Bone clefts numbered. (B) Soft tissue clefts numbered. Original artwork by the authors.

Tessier cleft number 11, or superomedial orbitofrontal cleft, is associated with ocular hypertelorism and coloboma of the medial third of the upper eyelid, sometimes extending through the eyebrow. At the level of bone tissue, a frontal encephalocele can be present in the forehead (Figure 58). In some cases, Tessier cleft number 11 is the cranial correspondent or even an extension of the facial Tessier cleft number 3.

References

David, D. J., M. H. Moore, and R. D. Cooter. 1989. "Tessier Clefts Revisited with a Third Dimension." *The Cleft Palate Journal* 26 (3): 163–84; discussion 184-5.

Tessier, Paul. 1976. "Anatomical Classification of Facial, Cranio-Facial and Latero-Facial Clefts." *Journal of Maxillofacial Surgery* 4: 69–92. https://doi.org/10.1016/s0301-0503(76)80013-6.

Winters, Ryan. 2016. "Tessier Clefts and Hypertelorism". *Facial Plastic Surgery Clinics of North America* 24 (4): 545–58. https://doi.org/10.1016/j.fsc.2016.06.013.

Tessier cleft number 11

Case 46

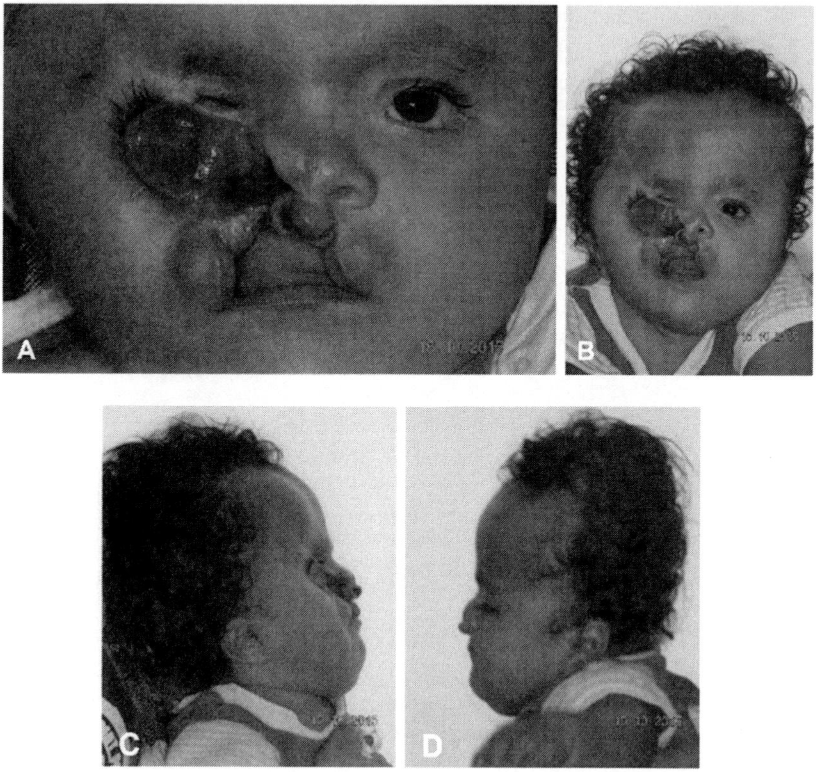

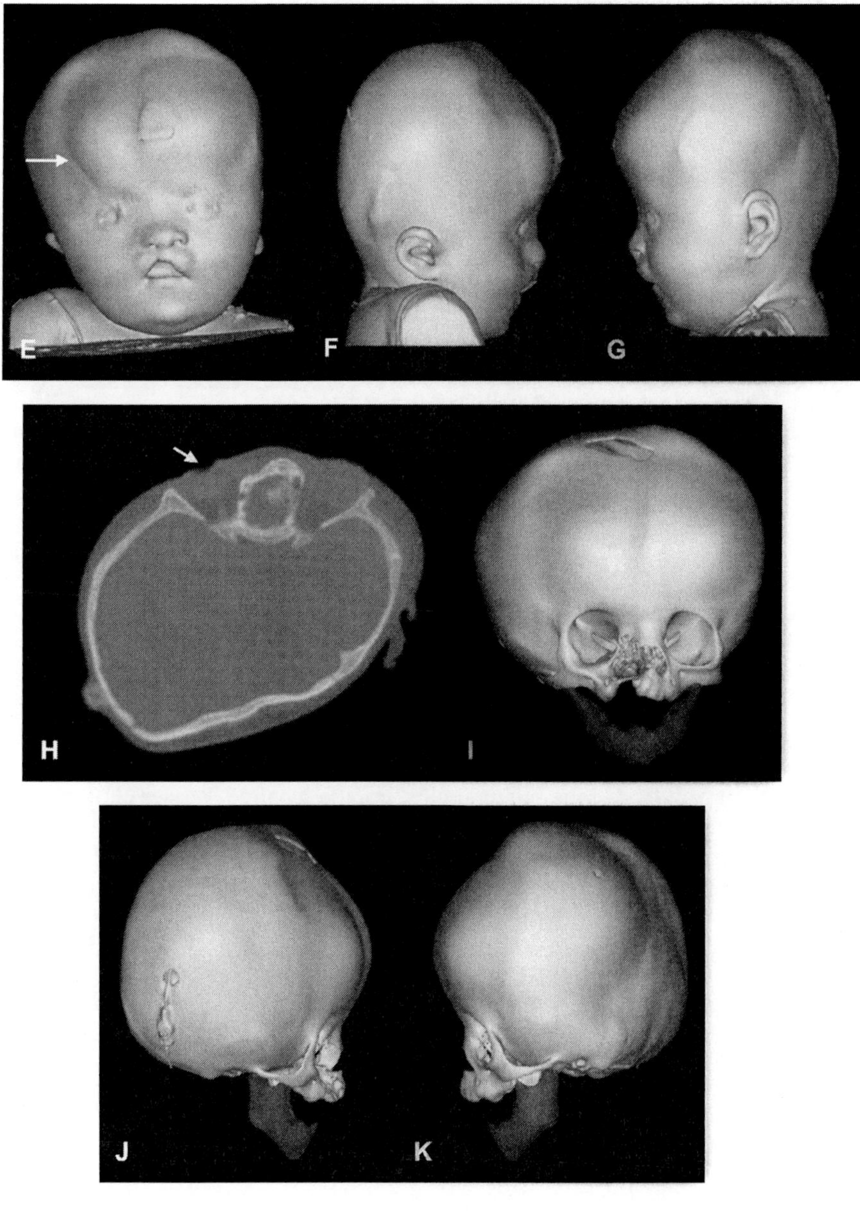
E
F
G
H
I
J
K

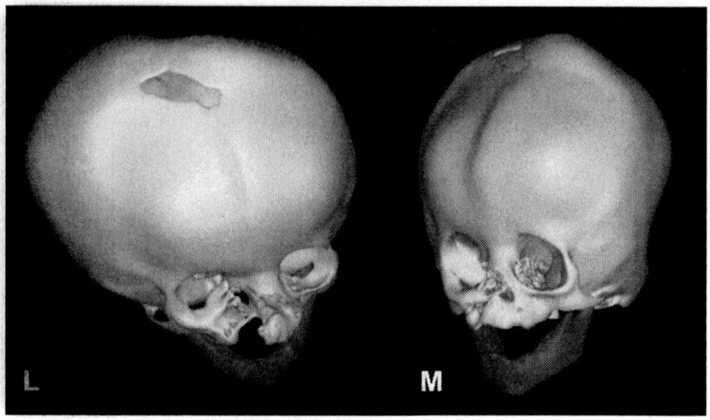

Figure 59– Male patient with a right Tessier cleft number 11 with amniotic band sequence. A-C: clinical phenotype at 11 months old. Note in the soft tissue the turricephaly, the broad forehead, the prominent metopic forehead, and a right superomedial orbital cleft involving the medial one-third upper eyelid and extending through the eyebrow to the frontal hairline (Tessier cleft number 11). Ocular hypertelorism and anophthalmia are observed. A wide right oro-nasal-ocular cleft (Tessier cleft number 3) disrupts the ocular development resulting in a failed palpebral structure, and a large ectopic palpebral tissue is seen in the face. A right lateral orbito-maxillary-oral cleft (Tessier cleft number 5) is also present. A right unilateral complete cleft lip and palate and a left cleft lip are also associated. E-M: computed tomography exam was obtained at 12 months old. Figures E to G show the clefts in soft tissue: the bilateral cleft lip, the repaired Tessier cleft number 3, and the Tessier cleft number 11 (arrow). Figure H is a CT axial section showing the ocular anomaly and craniofacial asymmetry. Figures I to M are 3D reconstructions of the hard tissue. Note the turricephaly; there is no bone cleft in the frontal region on the right or the right alveolar cleft and an absence of the medial maxillary wall (Tessier number 3). A right notch in the infraorbital rim (Tessier number 5) and bilateral hypoplasia of the zygomatic complex are observed.

CHAPTER THIRTEEN

TESSIER CLEFT NUMBER 12: THE MEDIAL FRONTOCRANIAL CLEFT

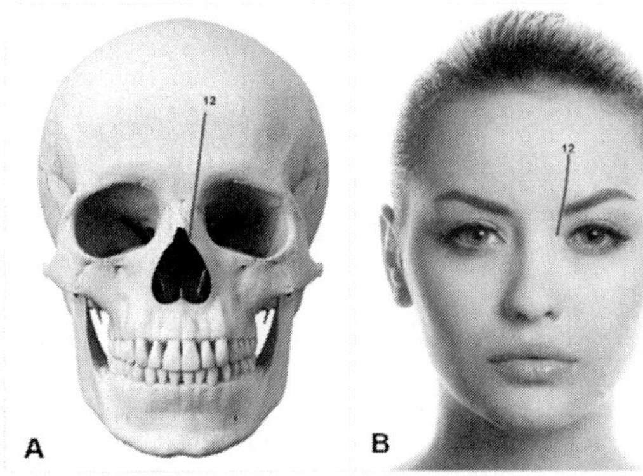

Figure 60– Localization of Tessier cleft number 12. (A) Bone clefts numbered. (B) Soft tissue clefts numbered. Original artwork by the authors.

Tessier cleft number 12, also called medial frontocranial cleft, is characterized by a flat frontal process with the cleft extending to the ethmoid bone. The frontal sinus is usually enlarged (Figure 60). The Tessier cleft number 12 represents the Tessier cleft number 2 in the cranium.

References

David, D. J., M. H. Moore, and R. D. Cooter. 1989. "Tessier Clefts Revisited with a Third Dimension." *The Cleft Palate Journal* 26 (3): 163–84; discussion 184-5.

Tessier, Paul. 1976. "Anatomical Classification of Facial, Cranio-Facial and Latero-Facial Clefts." *Journal of Maxillofacial Surgery* 4: 69–92. https://doi.org/10.1016/s0301-0503(76)80013-6.

Winters, Ryan. 2016. "Tessier Clefts and Hypertelorism". *Facial Plastic Surgery Clinics of North America* 24 (4): 545–58. https://doi.org/10.1016/j.fsc.2016.06.013.

Tessier cleft number 12

Case 47

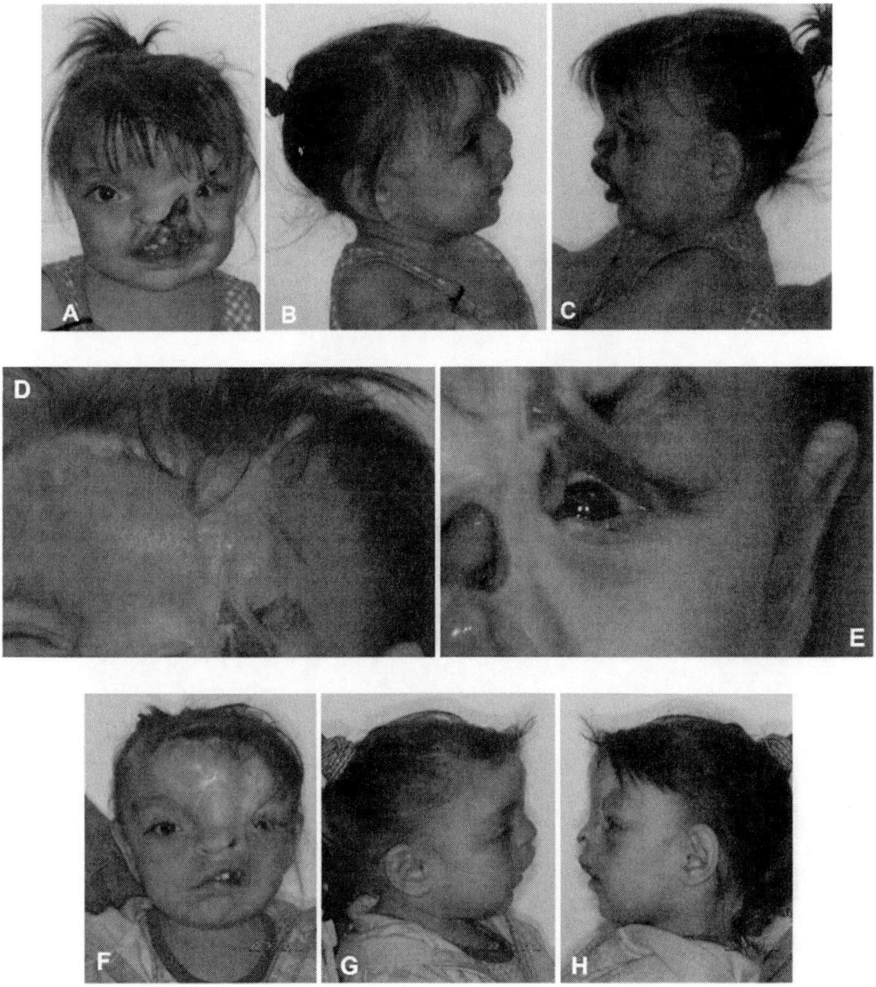

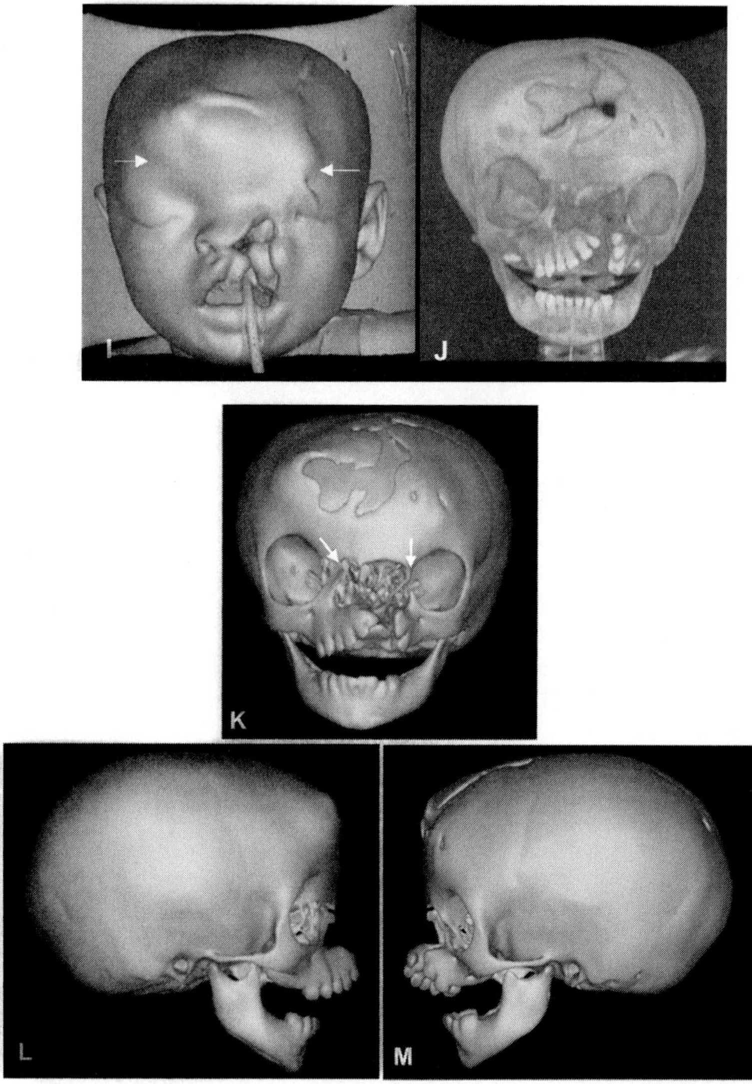
I
J
K
L
M

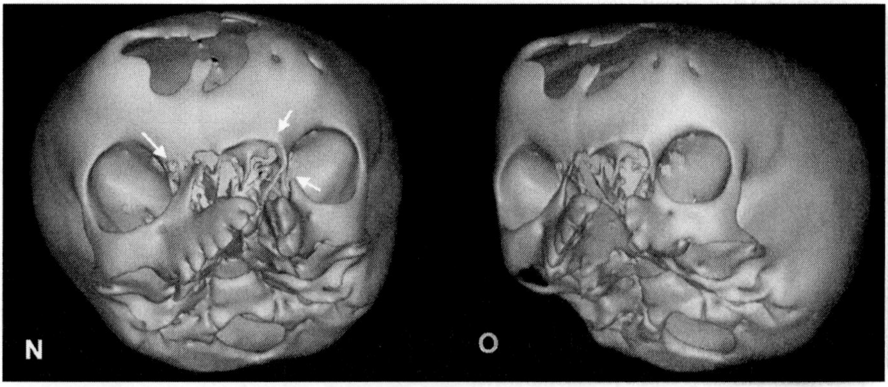

Figure 61 – female patient with a Tessier Cleft number 12 associated with amniotic bands sequence. A-E: clinical phenotype at one year and eight months years old. Note in the soft tissue the frontal prominence with a frontonasal encephalocele, an ocular hypertelorism, an abnormal upper eyelid with a left cleft and fusion with a frontal issue affecting the root eyebrow (Tessier cleft number 12). Observe a wide left cleft lip and palate extending superiorly to the lower eyelid's medial canthus (Tessier cleft number 3). F-H: clinical phenotype at two years and seven months showing the repaired clefts. I-O: computed tomography examination obtained at two years and one month old. Figure I shows an irregular frontonasal region, an abnormal upper left eyelid and a wide left oronasal and ocular cleft. Figure J is a translucent 3D view showing a wide bone failure in the frontonasal process and a wide left oronasal cleft with a protruded premaxilla. K-O: CT 3D reconstructions of bone tissue. Note the wide bone failure in the frontonasal process, the decreased left orbital size and a frontocranial cleft originating at the nasal bone and extending to the medial superior orbital rim (Tessier number 12) bilateral. A wide left oral cleft communicating with the wide nasal cavity and inner canthus of the orbital cavity (Tessier number 3) is also present. K: note in Figures L and M the protruded maxilla. The oblique views (Figure N, O) show a groove (arrow) in the median frontal line and a cleft in the nasal bone (arrow) communicating the orbit with the maxillary sinus and oral cavity (Tessier cleft number 3). K-L: panoramic and periapical radiograph at nine years old showing agenesis of the maxillary lateral incisors (22) on the left and maxillary alveolar defect between the central incisor and canine (21–23).

Case 48

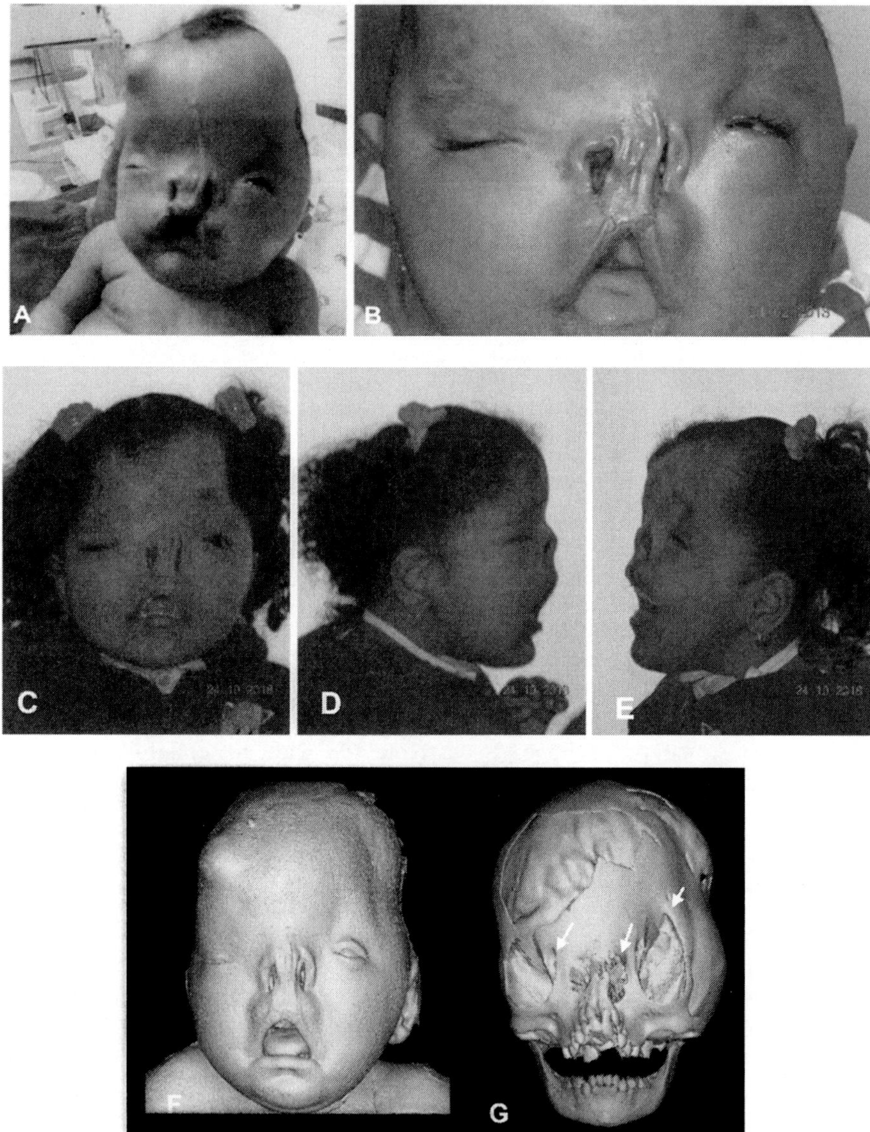

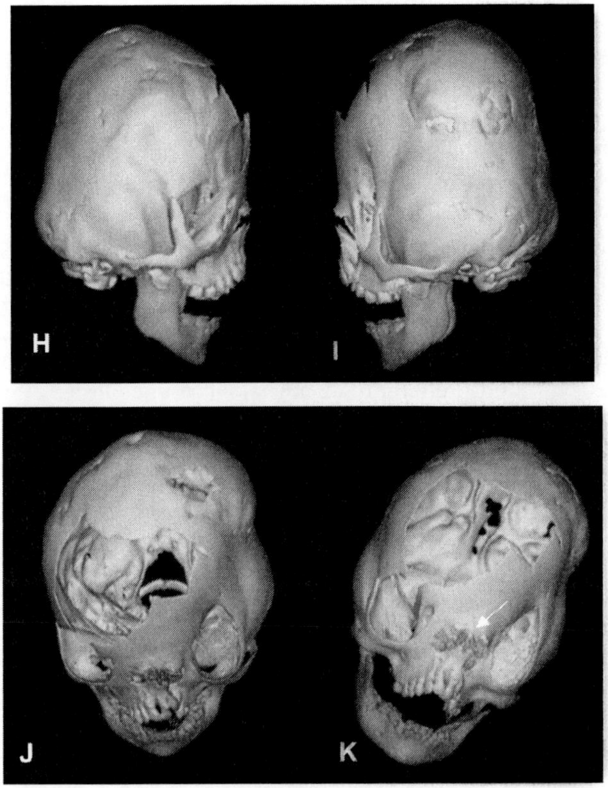

Figure 62 – Female patient with a Tessier cleft number 12 associated with amniotic band sequence. A-B: clinical phenotype at five months old. Note the turricephaly, a right encephalocele in the frontal bone, the absent eyebrows, severe ocular hypertelorism, the short palpebral fissures and the severe midface hypoplasia. A severe bifid nose with agenesis of the nasal bone and columella, a midline notch and a bilateral cleft lip associated with underdevelopment of the nasal alae (Tessier cleft number 2) were also present. Note that on the left side, a groove between the nasal and the ocular region extends to the superomedial orbital region, involving the medial one-third upper eyelid extending through the eyebrow to the frontal hairline (Tessier cleft number 11). C-E: facial photographs at five years old showing the repaired clefts. F-K: computed tomography examination obtained at three years old. In Figure F, note the right encephalocele in the frontal bone. Figures G to K are CT 3D reconstructions of the hard tissue. Note the turricephaly, the flattened frontal bone and the wide right bone failure in the

frontal bone affecting the superomedial orbital margin (Tessier cleft number 10). Bilateral wide orbital cavities, a cleft in the superomedial orbital margin (Tessier cleft number 10) and ocular hypertelorism were also present. Observe the abnormal nasal cavity with an ectopic premaxilla displaced to the nasal bridge medial portion. The nasal septum agenesis and a glabella extreme lateral displacement and increased distance between the olfactory grooves were present bilaterally (Tessier cleft number 2) and associated with Tessier cleft number 12 bilaterally. A midline cleft extending from the maxillary central incisors to the nasal cavity (Tessier cleft number 0) was present. Also, note the midface hypoplasia.

Case published in Tonello, Cristiano, Michele Madeira Brandão and Nivaldo Alonso. 2021. "Sinus Pericranii—Unusual Anatomic Obstacle to Posterior Decompression on an Amniotic Band Sequence". *Child's Nervous System: ChNS: Official Journal of the International Society for Pediatric Neurosurgery* 37 (4): 1369–72. https://doi.org/10.1007/s00381-020-04816-y.

.

Case 49

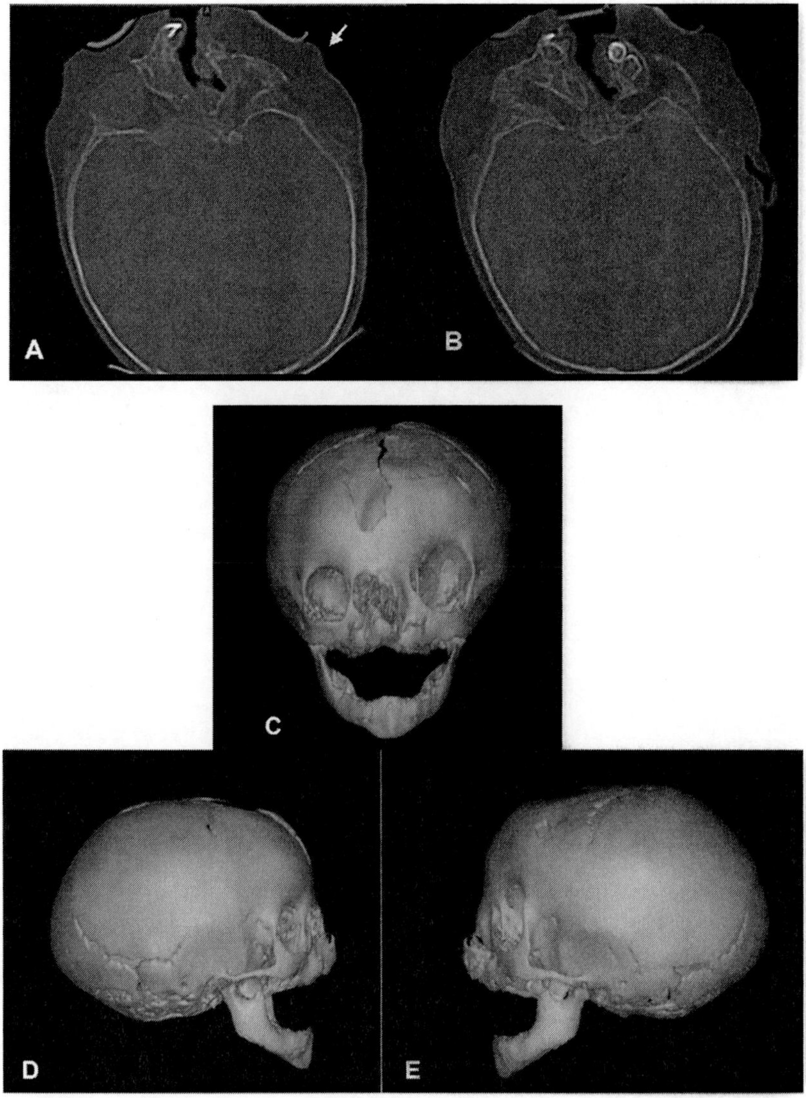

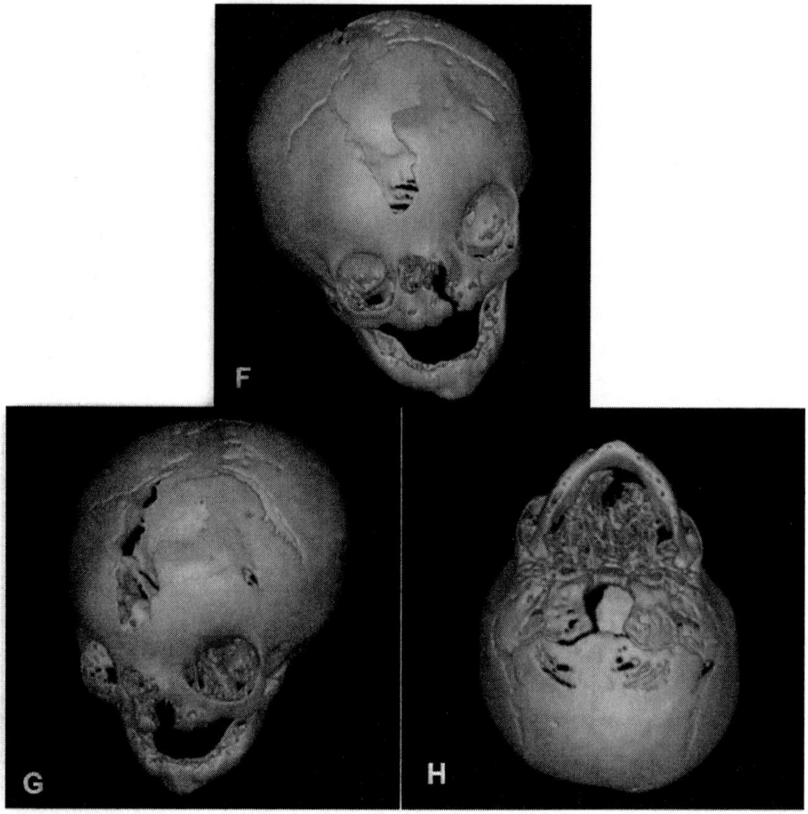

Figure 63 – Female patient with a Tessier Cleft number 12 with amniotic bands sequence. A-H: computed tomography exam obtained at five months old. Figure A shows a CT coronal section. Note the left microphthalmia/anophthalmia (arrow) and the left cleft lip and palate. Figures C to H reveal 3D CT 3D reconstructions of the hard tissue. Note the wide frontonasal bone failure, the ocular hypertelorism, the orbit asymmetry, the wide left orbital cavity, and a wide nasal cavity with notching in the nasal bones (Tessier cleft number 2) extending to the frontal bone (Tessier cleft number 12). The frontal process of the maxilla is flat (arrow in Figure E).

CHAPTER FOURTEEN

TESSIER CLEFT NUMBER 13: THE PARAMEDIAN FRONTAL CLEFT

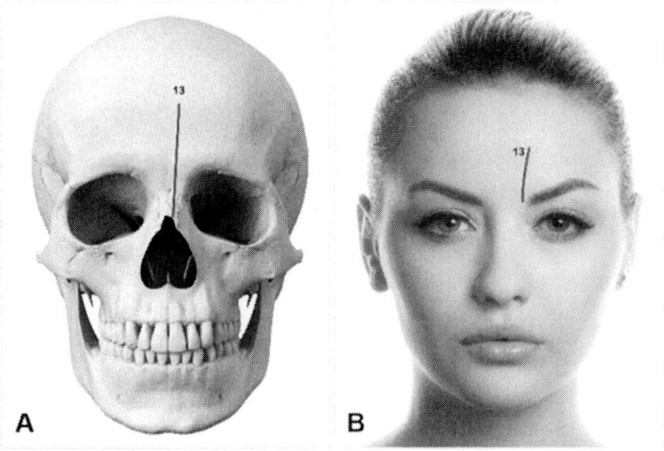

Figure 64 –Localization of Tessier cleft number 13. (A) Bone clefts numbered. (B) Soft tissue clefts numbered. Original artwork by the authors.

Tessier cleft number 13, or medial nasofrontal cleft, corresponds to the facial cleft number 1 and is located next to the midline of the nasal bone to the frontal region (Figure 64). In many cases, encephaloceles and ocular hypertelorism are associated.

References

David, D. J., M. H. Moore, and R. D. Cooter. 1989. "Tessier Clefts Revisited with a Third Dimension." *Cleft Palate J* 26 (3): 184–85.

Pellerin, Philippe. 2022. "Management of Hypertelorism". *Journal of Pediatric Neurosciences* 17 (5): 4. https://doi.org/10.4103/jpn.jpn_43_22.

Tessier, Paul. 1976. "Anatomical Classification of Facial, Cranio-Facial and Latero-Facial Clefts." *Journal of Maxillofacial Surgery* 4: 69–92. https://doi.org/10.1016/s0301-0503(76)80013-6.

Winters, Ryan. 2016. "Tessier Clefts and Hypertelorism". *Facial Plastic Surgery Clinics of North America* 24 (4): 545–58. https://doi.org/10.1016/j.fsc.2016.06.013.

Tessier cleft number 13

Case 50

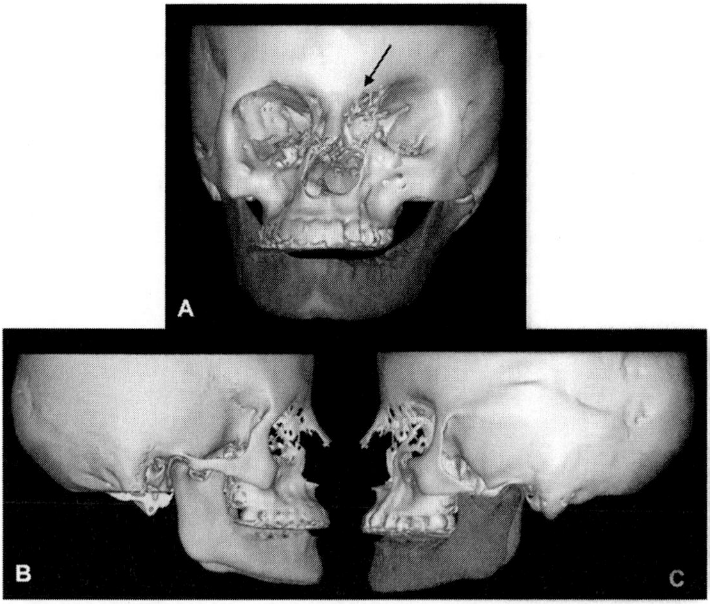

Figure 65 - *Image described in* Case 42. A-C: computed tomography exam taken at 16 years old displays a decreased orbital size on the left side. The nasal cavity is preserved, and the left bony failure in the nasal bone suggests Tessier cleft number 13 (arrow) is associated with a left superolateral orbital cleft extending to the temporal fossa (Tessier number 9). On the right side, an infraorbital rim hypoplastic suggests Tessier cleft number 6.

CHAPTER FIFTEEN

TESSIER CLEFT NUMBER 14: MIDLINE CRANIAL CLEFT

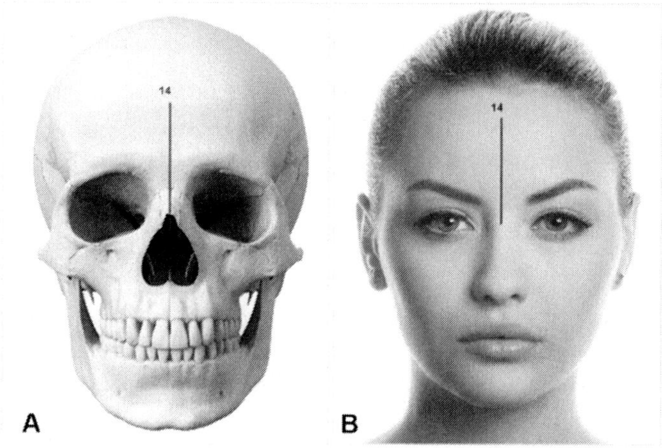

Figure 66 – Localization of Tessier cleft number 14. (A) Bone clefts numbered. (B) Soft tissue clefts numbered. Original artwork by the authors.

Tessier cleft number 14, the midline cranial cleft, is associated with a bifid nose corresponding to the facial cleft number 0 (Figure 66). Frontal encephalocele and ocular hypertelorism with frontal and glabella flattening are usually present.

References

David, D. J., M. H. Moore, and R. D. Cooter. 1989. "Tessier Clefts Revisited with a Third Dimension." *Cleft Palate J* 26 (3): 184–85.

Nam, S. M., and Y. B. Kim. 2014. "The Tessier Number 14 Facial Cleft: A 20-Year Follow-Up." *J Craniomaxillofac Surg* 42 (7): 1397–1401. https://doi.org/10.1016/j.jcms.2014.03.032

Pellerin, Philippe. 2022. "Management of Hypertelorism". *Journal of Pediatric Neurosciences* 17 (5): 4. https://doi.org/10.4103/jpn.jpn_43_22.

Tessier, Paul. 1976. "Anatomical Classification of Facial, Cranio-Facial and Latero-Facial Clefts." *Journal of Maxillofacial Surgery* 4: 69–92. https://doi.org/10.1016/s0301-0503(76)80013-6.

Winters, Ryan. 2016. "Tessier Clefts and Hypertelorism". *Facial Plastic Surgery Clinics of North America* 24 (4): 545–58. https://doi.org/10.1016/j.fsc.2016.06.013.

Tessier cleft number 14

Case 51

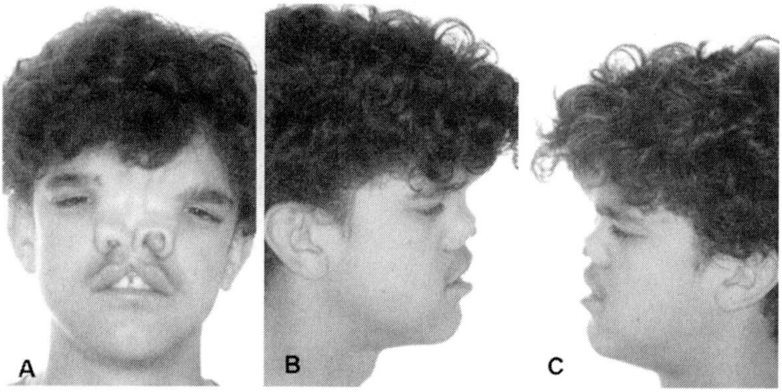

Case 6 published in: Guion-Almeida, Maria Leine, Cecília Mellado, Constanza Beltrán and A. Richieri-Costa. 2007. "Pai Syndrome: Report of Seven South American Patients". *American Journal of Medical Genetics. Part A* 143A (24): 3273–79. https://doi.org/10.1002/ajmg.a.31962.

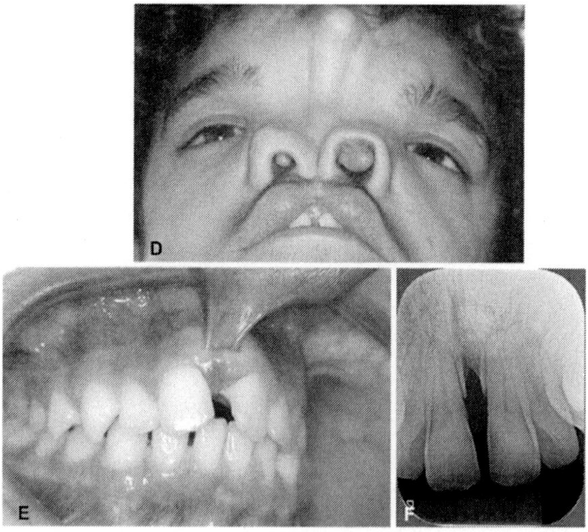

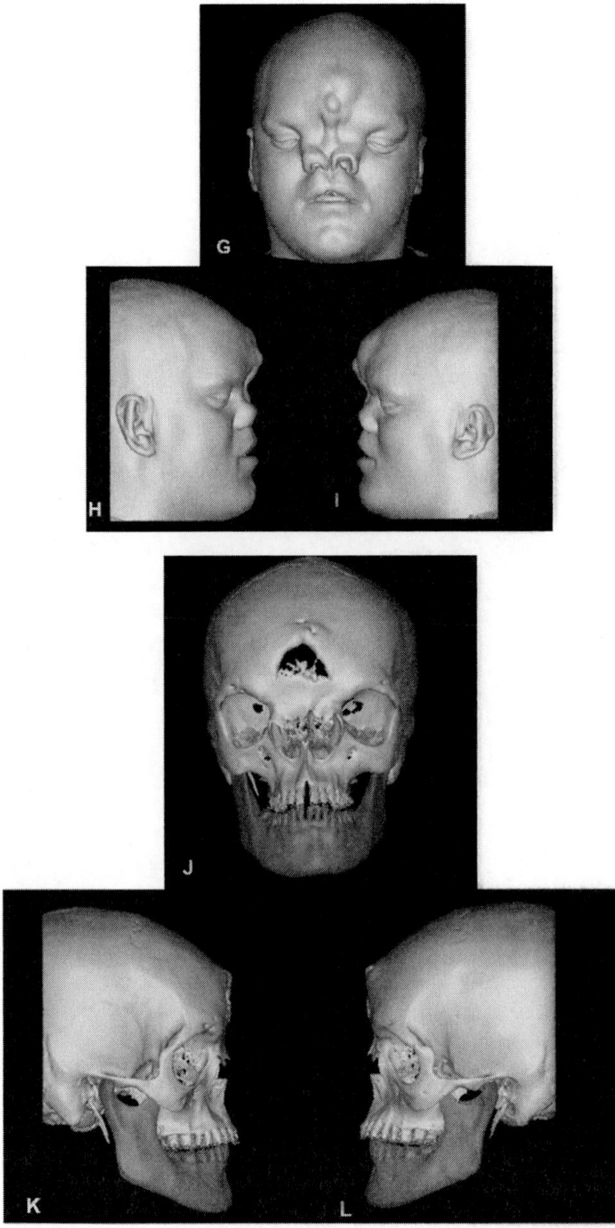
G
H
I
J
K
L

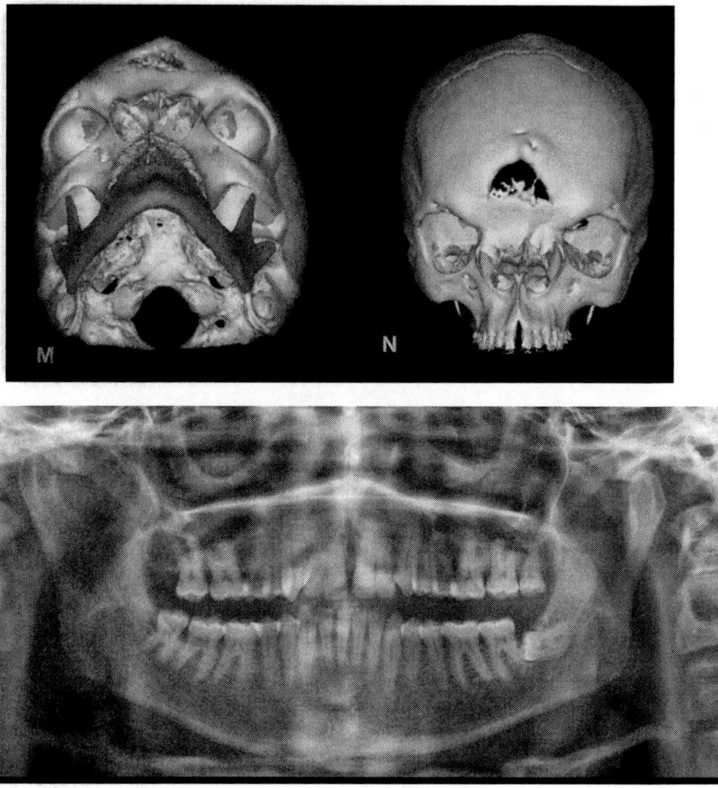

Figure 67 – Male patient with Tessier cleft number 14 and Pai syndrome. A-E: clinical phenotype at 15 years old. Note the wide forehead, an abnormal frontal hairline, a midline frontal encephalocele and severe ocular hypertelorism. A bifid nose with no nasal bridge and a wide nostril with cutaneous polyps were present. A midline cleft lip (close-up in Figure D) and midface hypoplasia were also seen. Figure E shows a bifid frenulum of the upper lip and a midline diastema in the maxillary dental arch. F: periapical radiograph showing a midline maxillary alveolar cleft. G-N: computed tomography exams were obtained at 27 years old. In Figure G, note in the soft tissue a frontal bossing with midline encephalocele, a wide midline cleft lip along a bifid nose and the ocular hypertelorism until the encephalocele (Tessier cleft numbers 0 to 14). The lateral views demonstrate midface hypoplasia. Figures J to N are CT 3D reconstructions of the hard tissue showing a prominent upper orbital bridge, a groove in the sphenoid bone and a duplicated nasal bone. Observe the widened nasal

cavity associated with the bifid nose and the abnormal nasal structure resembling a nasal duplication. A nasal cleft (Tessier number 12) was also present. In Figure M, note the nasal septum agenesis and the glabella with an extreme lateral displacement. An increased distance between the olfactory grooves was present. In Figure N, observe the midline cranial cleft (Tessier cleft number 14), the frontal bone abnormally flat with a large midline defect. O: panoramic radiograph at 29 years old shows no dental anomalies and median alveolar defects between the central incisors.

CHAPTER SIXTEEN

TESSIER CLEFT NUMBER 30: THE MANDIBULAR CLEFT

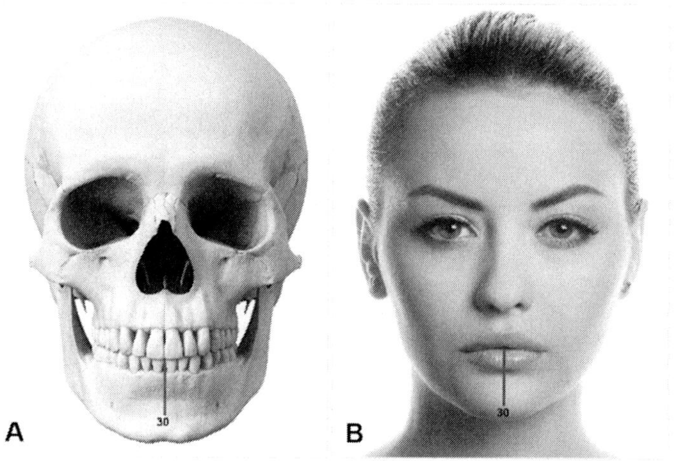

Figure 68 – Localization of Tessier cleft number 30. (A) Bone clefts numbered. (B) Soft tissue clefts numbered. Original artwork by the authors.

Tessier cleft number 30, or the mandibular cleft, occurs in the lower lip or the mandibular alveolar arch (Figure 68). This cleft occurs due to a fusion and ossification failure of the mandibular processes. Adherence of the tongue on the buccal floor or cleft of the tongue that varies from the anterior bifid tip with ankyloglossia to the bony cleft margins or marked tongue hypoplasia and cleft extension to the cervical region can also be observed in association with the mandibular cleft.

References

Armstrong, A. P., and N. Waterhouse. 1996. "Tessier 30 Median Mandibular Cleft: Case Report and Literature Review." *Br J Plast Surg* 49 (8): 536–38. https://doi.org/ 10.1016/s0007-1226(96)90130-7

David, D. J., M. H. Moore, and R. D. Cooter. 1989. "Tessier Clefts Revisited with a Third Dimension." *The Cleft Palate Journal* 26 (3): 163–84; discussion 184-5.

Favaro, F. P., R. M. Zechi-Ceide, and C. W. Alvarez. 2011. "Richieri-Costa-Pereira Syndrome: A Unique Acrofacial Dysostosis Type. An Overview of the Brazilian Cases." *Am J Med Genet A* 155 (2): 322–31. https://doi.org/ 10.1002/ajmg.a.33806.

Hennekam, Raoul, Judith E. Allanson, and Ian Krantz. 2010. *Gorlin's Syndromes of the Head and Neck*. 5th ed. New York, NY: Oxford University Press.

Ladani, P., H. F. Sailer, and R. Sabnis. 2013. "Tessier 30 Symphyseal Mandibular Cleft: Early Simultaneous Soft and Hard Tissue Correction - a Case Report." *J Craniomaxillofac Surg* 41 (8): 735–39. https://doi.org/10.1016/j.jcms.2012.12.009.

Tafreshi, Mona, Soroosh Aminolsharieh Najafi, Reyhaneh Hasheminejad, Arezoo Mirfazeli and Akbar Shafiee. 2015. "Tessier Number 30 Clefts with Congenital Heart Defects." *Iranian Red Crescent Medical Journal* 17 (3). https://doi.org/10.5812/ircmj.19078.

Tessier, Paul. 1976. "Anatomical Classification of Facial, Cranio-Facial and Latero-Facial Clefts." *Journal of Maxillofacial Surgery* 4: 69–92. https://doi.org/10.1016/s0301-0503(76)80013-6.

Tonello, Cristiano, Ines Correia Pinto de Matos, Leonardo Bezerra Feitosa, Adriano Porto Peixoto and Nivaldo Alonso. 2021. "Congenital Midline Cervical Cleft: A Variant of Tessier Number 30 Cleft Causing Micrognathia." *The Cleft Palate-Craniofacial Journal: Official Publication of the American Cleft Palate-Craniofacial Association* 58 (11): 1446–51. https://doi.org/10.1177/1055665620987412.

Tessier, Paul. 1976. "Anatomical Classification of Facial, Cranio-Facial and Latero-Facial Clefts." *Journal of Maxillofacial Surgery* 4: 69–92. https://doi.org/10.1016/s0301-0503(76)80013-6.

Winters, Ryan. 2016. "Tessier Clefts and Hypertelorism". *Facial Plastic Surgery Clinics of North America* 24 (4): 545–58. https://doi.org/10.1016/j.fsc.2016.06.013.

Tessier cleft number 30

Case 52

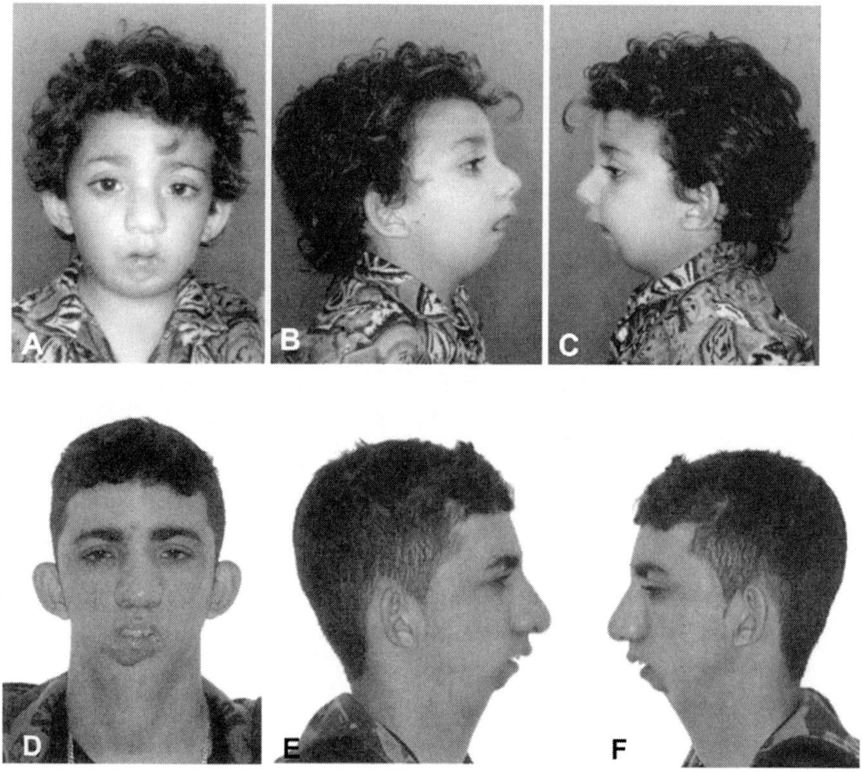

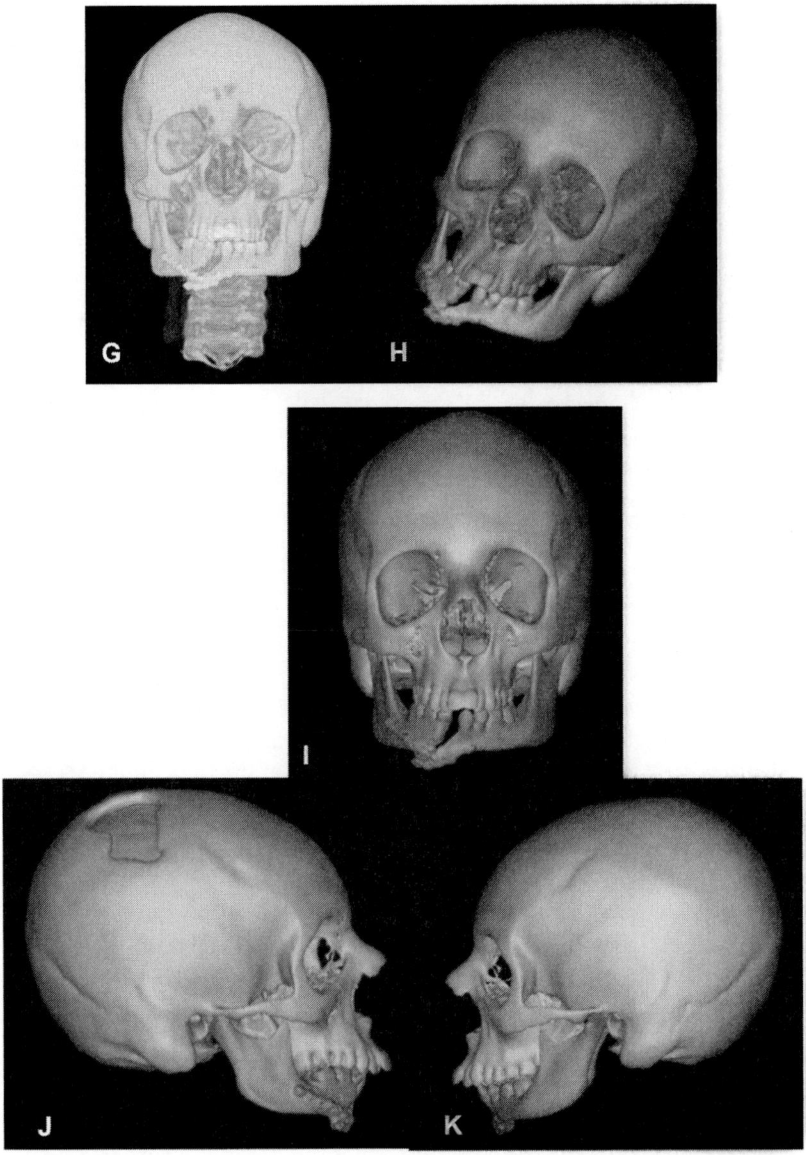
G
H
I
J
K

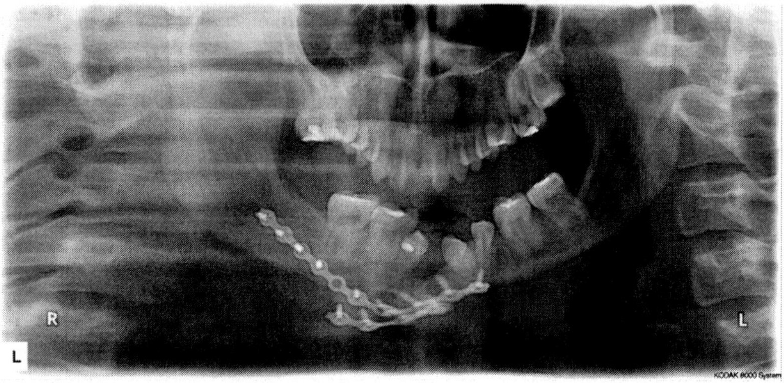

Figure 69– Male patient with a Tessier cleft number 30 associated with Richieri-Costa-Pereira syndrome (OMIM 268305). A-C: clinical phenotype at three years old. Note the prominent nose, the microstomia, the severe retromicrognathia and the low-set and prominent ears. D-F: clinical phenotype at 19 years old showing extreme retromicrognathia. G-K: computed tomography examination obtained at ten years old. Figure G is a translucent CT 3D view showing the wide median mandibular cleft (Tessier cleft number 30). Figures H to K are CT 3D reconstructions of the hard tissue. Note the wide median mandibular cleft without the mandibular central and lateral incisors. L: panoramic radiograph at ten years old showing multiple tooth agenesis bilateral central and lateral incisors (32, 31, 41 and 42), canine (43) and first premolar (44) on the right and the second premolar (35).

Published in: Favaro, Francine Pinheiro, Roseli Maria Zechi-Ceide, Camila Wenceslau Alvarez, Luciana P. Maximino, Luis Fernando B. B. Antunes, Antonio Richieri-Costa and Maria Leine Guion-Almeida. 2011. "Richieri-Costa-Pereira Syndrome: A Unique Acrofacial Dysostosis Type. An Overview of the Brazilian Cases". *American Journal of Medical Genetics. Part A* 155 (2): 322–31. https://doi.org/10.1002/ajmg.a.33806.

(Patient 10).

Case 53

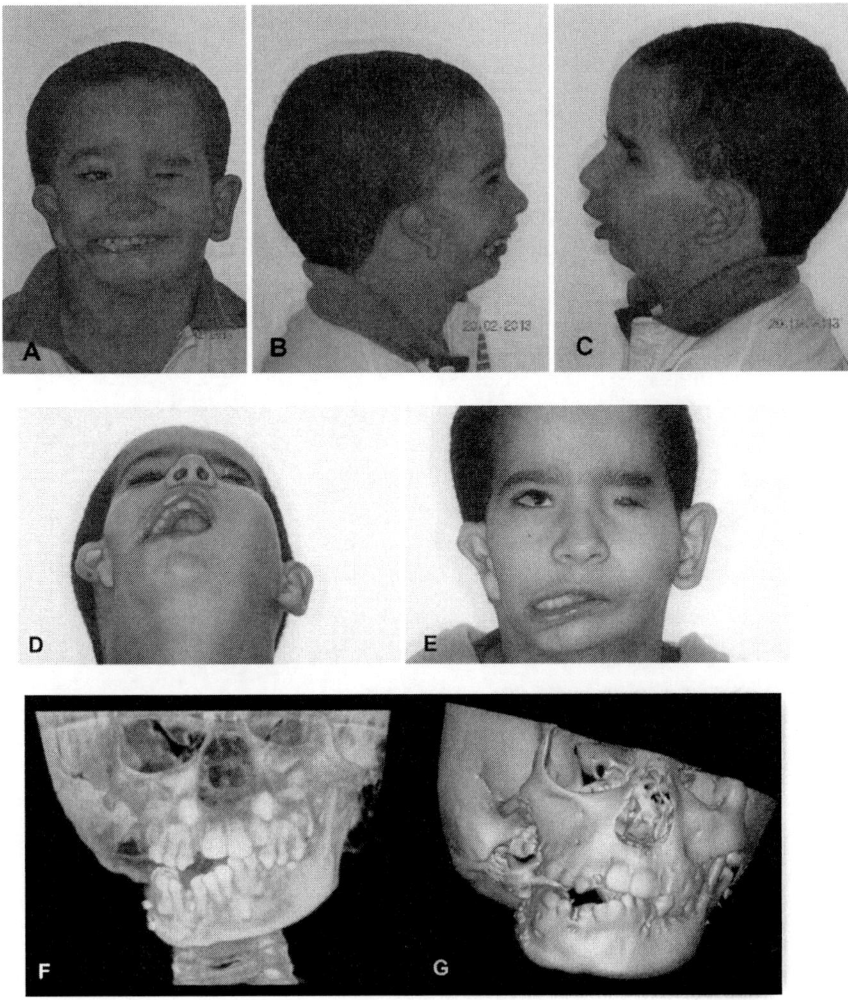

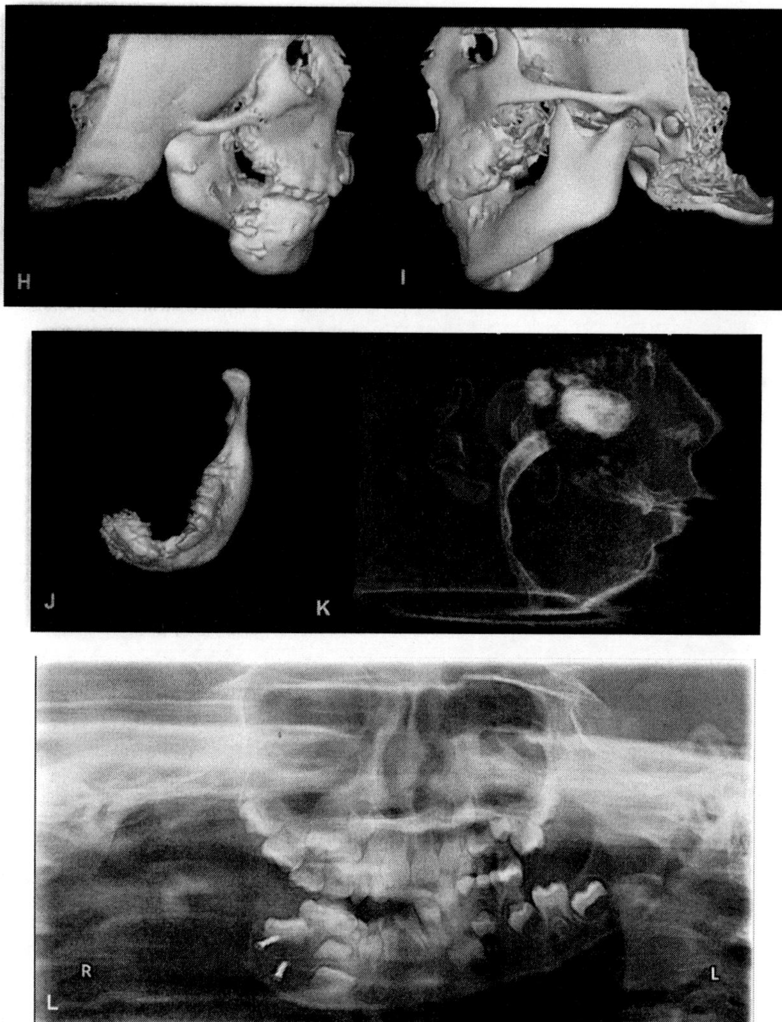

Published in Vendramini-Pittoli, Siulan, Maria L. Guion-Almeida, Juliana M. Santos, Silvio M. Garcia Júnior, Mauricio M. Yoshida, Antonio Richieri-Costa and Nancy M. Kokitsu-Nakata. 2015. “An Unusual Presentation of Oculoauriculovertebral Spectrum with a Tessier 30 Cleft: Report on Two Cases: Report on Two Cases". *Clinical Dysmorphology* 24 (4): 144–50. https://doi.org/10.1097/MCD.0000000000000085 (Case 1).

Figure 70 – Male patient with a Tessier number 30 cleft associated with the oculoauriculovertebral spectrum. A-C: clinical phenotype at four years old. Note the facial asymmetry, the left microphthalmia and the right lateral Tessier number 7 cleft. Type II microtia with external auditory canal atresia on the right side and midline cleft of the lower lip with a mandibular asymmetry (Tessier 30 cleft) were seen. D-E: clinical phenotype at nine years old. Observe in Figure E the epibulbar dermoid and the mandibular asymmetry. F-K: computed tomography examination obtained postoperatively at one year and eight months old. Figure F is a translucent 3D view of the hard tissue showing the mandibular cleft. Figures G to I are CT 3D reconstructions of the hard tissue. Note the left decreased orbital size, the facial asymmetry, the right short and hypoplastic zygomatic arch and the right deficiency of the zygomatic process of the temporal bone. Figure J shows the mandibular cleft and the agenesis of the mandibular ramus and glenoid fossa, condyle and coronoid process on the right side. Figure K demonstrates a narrow upper airway. L: panoramic radiograph at six years old shows no dental anomalies.

Case 54

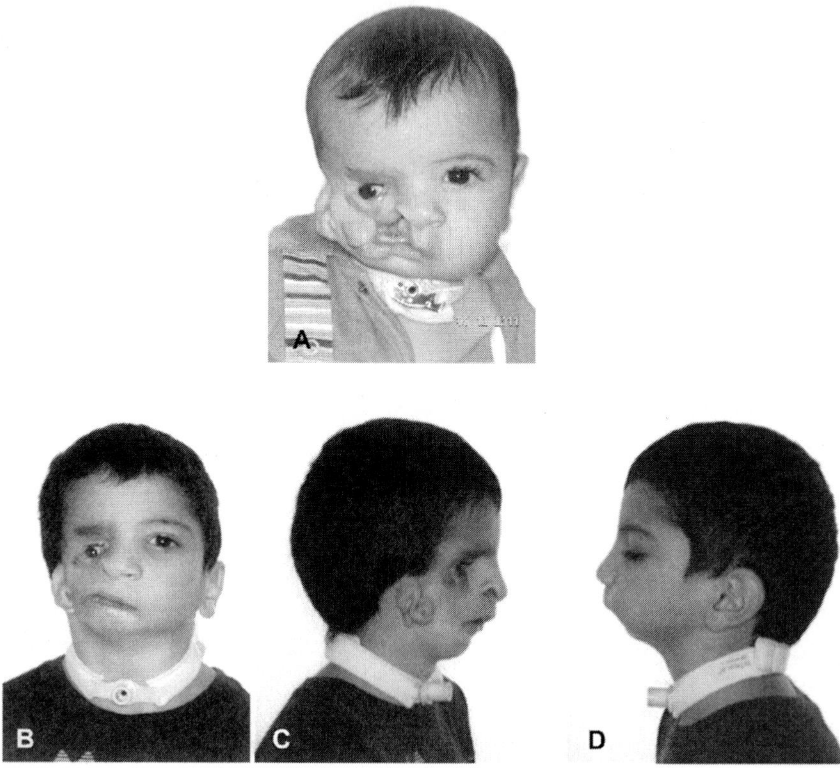

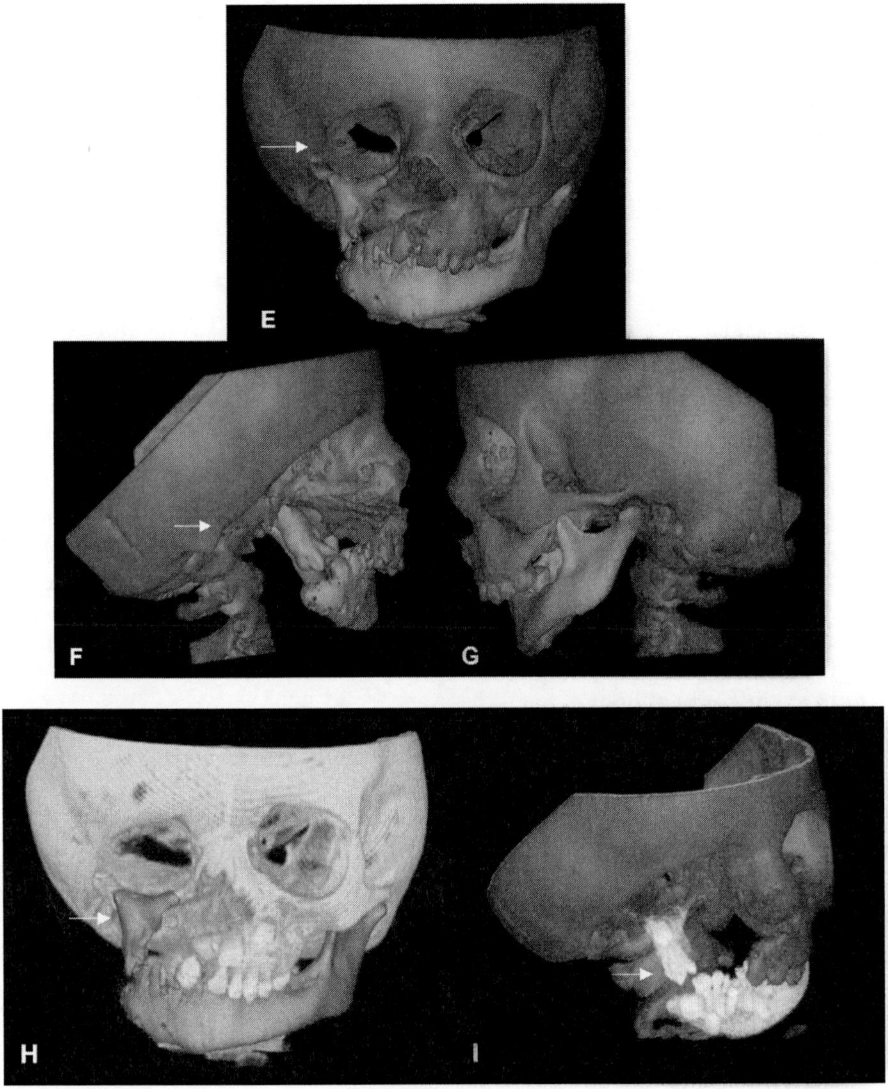

Figure 71 – Male patient with a Tessier number 30 cleft associated with the oculoauriculovertebral spectrum. A: clinical phenotype at three months old. Note the ocular hypertelorism, the severe facial asymmetry and the classical cleft lip and palate associated with complex facial clefts on the right side. Observe also the sparse right eyebrow and upper eyelashes (Tessier cleft

number 9), a true lateral eyelid coloboma with the absence of the outer canthus (Tessier cleft number 8), a right lateral cleft (Tessier cleft number 7). A wide right orofacial cleft with an absence of an alveolar arch from the central incisors until the premolar region extending to the frontal process of the maxilla, lacrimal fossa orbit, nose, and full lower eyelid (Tessier cleft numbers 3 and 4) were present. A wide right cleft also extended to the medial region of the oral commissure across the cheek as a furrow until the lower eyelid was seen (Tessier cleft number 5). Note the mandibular cleft (Tessier cleft number 30) and the type III microtia with external auditory canal agenesis. B-D: clinical phenotype at five years old showing the repaired clefts. E-G: computed tomography obtained postoperatively at five years old. Note the decreased right orbital size, the broad nasal cavity, and the frontozygomatic bony cleft producing the absence of the lateral orbital rim (Tessier cleft number 8). The right temporozygomatic cleft was associated with complete agenesis of the zygomatic arch and severe mandibular hypoplasia with agenesis of the ramus, condyle, coronoid process, and glenoid fossa (Tessier cleft number 7). On the right side, the agenesis of a wide portion of the maxilla and the zygomatic complex with communication with the orbit (Tessier cleft numbers 6, 5 and 4) are notable. Also, observe the cleft in the right maxillary sinus and nose (Tessier cleft number 3) and a right mandibular cleft (Tessier cleft number 30). Figures H to I are translucent 3D views showing a vestigial maxillary structure linked to the infraorbital floor.

Published in Vendramini-Pittoli, Siulan, Maria L. Guion-Almeida, Juliana M. Santos, Silvio M. Garcia Júnior, Mauricio M. Yoshida, Antonio Richieri-Costa and Nancy M. Kokitsu-Nakata. 2015. “An Unusual Presentation of Oculoauriculovertebral Spectrum with a Tessier 30 Cleft: Report on Two Cases: Report on Two Cases". *Clinical Dysmorphology* 24 (4): 144–50. https://doi.org/10.1097/MCD.0000000000000085 (Case 2).

CHAPTER SEVENTEEN

CRANIOFACIAL ANOMALIES: AN OVERALL VISION

Craniofacial anomalies are among the most common human anomalies. About one-third of newborns with congenital anomalies involve craniofacial structures, including fusion failure of the cranial bones, frontonasal dysplasia, first and second pharyngeal arches defects, and orofacial clefts. Consequently, it can affect other structures such as the central nervous system, eyes, nose, mouth, teeth and ears, compromising functions such as vision, hearing, breathing, feeding, communication and neuropsychological development. Each one of the craniofacial anomalies can occur isolated or as part of several syndromes, which usually involve multiple systems, representing a great challenge to the diagnosis, treatment, and prevention (Hennekam, Allanson and Krantz, 2010; Sanske, 2010, Ornoy 2020). Therefore, a rehabilitation team must include the integration of a multidisciplinary team, which includes clinicians, surgeons, dentists, otorhinolaryngologists, speech therapists, psychologists, physiotherapists and geneticists, among others. The first approach is the primary surgery, performed by craniofacial surgeons; however, the challenge to other professionals, who aim to develop new treatment methods and protocols to rehabilitate craniofacial anomalies in a multidisciplinary team, is far greater (Sanske, 2010).

The normal craniofacial development of vertebrates is a complex and dynamic process that involves the interaction between tissues derived from the ectoderm, mesoderm and endoderm, as well as the neural crest, also known as the fourth germ layer (Wilkie and Morris-Kay, 2001; Sanke, 2010; Szabo-Rogers et al. 2010; Twigg and Wilkie, 2015). The central nervous system (CNS) arises from the neural plate, a homogeneous layer of epithelial cells. The neural plate folds to form the neural tube and the enlarged anterior end segments into three vesicles. These vesicles are the developmental primordia of the forebrain (prosencephalon), midbrain (mesencephalon), and hindbrain (rhombencephalon). The expansion of the forebrain gives rise to the frontonasal process and the neural crest cells derived from the midbrain and hindbrain (Chai et al., 2000; Wilkie and Morris-kay, 2001; Mao and Nah, 2004). The central key to craniofacial development is the neural crest cells (NCC), which migrate from the rostral portion of the neural tube to populate the frontonasal region and the pharyngeal arches (Francis-West et al. 1998; Wilkie and Morris-kay, 2001; Passos-Bueno, 2009, Twigg and Wilkie, 2015; Roth et al. 2021). Both inductive and signalling activities coordinate the facial primordium growth from undifferentiated mesenchymal buds to an intricate mosaic of bone and cartilaginous structures that, combined with muscles and other tissues, will constitute the definitive face (Francis-West et al. 1998; Wilkie and Morris-kay, 2001; Alappat et al. 2003; Passos-Bueno, 2009). The complex interactions between multiple embryonic tissues, including the neural crest, the prechordal mesoderm and the ectoderm, require precise regulation of migration, growth, modelling, and differentiation of craniofacial tissues (Francis-West et al. 1998; Wilkie and Morris-Kay et al. 2001; Nancy, 2003; Jiang et al. 2006; Nie et al. 2006; Twigg and Wilkie, 2015). Disruption in the regulation of the craniofacial development process, caused by genetic or environmental factors, can result in different types of craniofacial anomalies (Francis-West et al. 1998; Wilkie and Morris-Kay et al. 2001; Jiang et al. 2006; Nie et al., 2006; Twigg and Wilkie, 2015; Ji et al. 2020), which mainly include structural CNS abnormalities, skull bone closure defects, craniofacial midline anomalies with ocular hypotelorism (holoprosencephaly) or with ocular hypertelorism (frontonasal process dysplasia), typical and atypical orofacial clefts, and first and second pharyngeal arches defects ((Wilkie and Morriss-Kay 2001; Hennekam, Allanson and Krantz, 2010; Casale and Giwa 2022). Morphological studies in animal models (natural or mutations modified by the action of teratogens and genes) and clinical, cytogenetic (identification of candidate loci), and molecular (direct linkage and sequencing studies) studies of human craniofacial anomalies have allowed us to understand some events of complex craniofacial development and to identify genes that regulate normal craniofacial development, including those encoding transcription factors, growth factors, growth factor receptors, and signalling molecules (Francis-West et al. 1998; Cobourne, 2000; Wilkie and Morris-Kay et al. 2001; Jiang, Bush and Lidral 2006; Nie et al. 2006, Cohen 2006; Passos-Bueno et al. 2009; Ciurea and Toader, 2009; Gordon et al. 2015; Twigg and Wilkie, 2015)

Orofacial Clefts: Clinical and Genetic Aspects

Orofacial clefts are the most common craniofacial congenital anomaly, with a prevalence of approximately 1:700, varying in relation to race and gender. The orofacial cleft can be subclassified into typical and atypical (or rare) clefts. The typical orofacial cleft includes cleft lip (CL) when it affects only the lip; cleft lip and palate (CLP) when it affects the lip and palate; and cleft palate (CP), when it affects only the palate (Rahimov, Jugessur, Murray 2012; Leslie and Marazita 2013; Worley, Patel and Kilpatrick 2018). The aetiology of the typical orofacial cleft is complex, caused by genes, the environment, or complex interaction between both (Lidral, Moreno and Bullard, 2008; Worley, Patel and Kilpatrick, 2018).

According to Fogh-Andersen (1942), in his classic work, the cleft lip, with or without palate involvement (CL/P), is genetic and embryologically distinct from a cleft palate without lip involvement (CP). Like other craniofacial anomalies, CL/P and CP can occur in syndromic and nonsyndromic forms. It has been observed that about 30% of CLP and 50% of CP cases are syndromic, many of them with genetic aetiology. More than 500 known syndromes include in their phenotypic spectrum the typical orofacial cleft; among these syndromes, the most common diagnoses include the Van der Woude syndrome (OMIM 119300), Stickler syndrome (OMIM108300), Velocardiofacial syndrome/del 22q11.2 deletion syndrome (OMIM 192430), ectrodactyly, ectodermal dysplasia and cleft lip/palate syndrome (OMIM 604292), and Treacher Collins syndrome (OMIM 154500 type 1, OMIM 248390 type 2, OMIM 613717 type 3 and OMIM 602000 type 4) (Murray, 2002; Lidral, Moreno and Bullard, 2008; Dixon et al. 2011; Johnson et al. 2011; Rahimov, Jugessur, Murray 2012; Wójcicki, Koźlik, Wójcicka 2016; Worley, Patel, Kilpatrick 2018). Other conditions with a typical orofacial cleft are rare, extremely rare, or a unique condition described in one case or family (Hennekam, Allanson and Krantz, 2010; Wieczorek, 2013; Setó-Salvia and Stanier, 2014; Gordon et al. 2015).

Despite the technological advances in genetics and genomics knowledge, the aetiology of the nonsyndromic orofacial cleft is unclear. It has been largely accepted that the orofacial cleft has a multifactorial inheritance, i.e., a combination of genetic and environmental factors (Murray, 2002; Hennekam, Allanson and Krantz, 2010, Leslie and Marazita, 2013, Worley, Patel and Kilpatrick 2018; Reynolds et al. 2020). Environmental factors include exposure to maternal smoking and maternal alcohol, which increase the risk for cleft lip and palate, while folate supplementation could prevent recurrences of cleft lip with or without cleft palate in families (Dixon et al.

2011; Krauss and Hong 2016). In relation to genetic influence, candidate genes or genome-wide association studies have found an association with cleft lips, the palate and genes *IRF6, TGFA, FGFR1, FGFR2, FOXE1, MTHFR, PDGFC, PVLR1, FGF8, MSX1, BMP4, SUMO, ARHGAP29* and *TP63*, among others (Tettamanti et al. 2017; Martinelli et al. 2020; Reynolds et al. 2020; Ji et al. 2021; Awotoye et al. 2022). Some loci, including the gene desert region on chromosome 8q24, and other chromosomes region, such as 9q21, 10q25 and 17q22, have also been proposed (Dixon et al. 2011, Leslie and Marazita 2013; Leslie et al. 2017, Tettamanti et al. 2017; Reynolds et al. 2020).

References

Alappat, Sylvia, Zun Yi Zhang and Yi Ping Chen. 2003. "Msx Homeobox Gene Family and Craniofacial Development." *Cell Research* 13 (6): 429–42. https://doi.org/10.1038/sj.cr.7290185.

Awotoye, W., C. Comnick, C. Pendleton, E. Zeng, A. Alade, P. A. Mossey, L. J. J. Gowans, et al. 2022. "Genome-Wide Gene-by-Sex Interaction Studies Identify Novel Nonsyndromic Orofacial Clefts Risk Locus." *Journal of Dental Research* 101 (4): 465–72. https://doi.org/10.1177/00220345211046614.

Casale, J., and A. O. Giwa. 2022. "Branchial Arches." *StatPearls [Internet]. Treasure Island (FL)*.

Chai, Y., X. Jiang, Y. Ito, P. Bringas, J. Han, D. H. Rowitch, P. Soriano, A. P. McMahon, and H. M. Sucov. 2000. "Fate of the Mammalian Cranial Neural Crest during Tooth and Mandibular Morphogenesis." *Development (Cambridge, England)* 127 (8): 1671–79. https://doi.org/10.1242/dev.127.8.1671.

Ciurea, Alexandru Vlad and Corneliu Toader. 2009. "Genetics of Craniosynostosis: Review of the Literature." *Journal of Medicine and Life* 2 (1): 5–17.

Cobourne, Martyn T. 2000. "Construction for the Modern Head: Current Concepts in Craniofacial Development." *Journal of Orthodontics* 27 (4): 307–14. https://doi.org/10.1093/ortho/27.4.307.

Cohen, M. Michael. 2006. *Perspectives on the Face*. New York, NY: Oxford University Press.

Dixon, Michael J., Mary L. Marazita, Terri H. Beaty, and Jeffrey C. Murray. 2011. "Cleft Lip and Palate: Understanding Genetic and Environmental Influences." *Nature Reviews. Genetics* 12 (3): 167–78. https://doi.org/10.1038/nrg2933.

Fogh-Andersen, P. 1942. *Inheritance of Harelip and Cleft Palate.* Copenhagen: Busck.

Gordon, Christopher T., K. Nicole Weaver, Roseli Maria Zechi-Ceide, Erik C. Madsen, Andre L. P. Tavares, Myriam Oufadem, Yukiko Kurihara, et al. 2015. "Mutations in the Endothelin Receptor Type A Cause Mandibulofacial Dysostosis with Alopecia." *The American Journal of Human Genetics* 96 (4): 519–31. https://doi.org/10.1016/j.ajhg.2015.01.015.

Hennekam, Raoul, Judith E. Allanson, and Ian Krantz. 2010. *Gorlin's Syndromes of the Head and Neck.* 5th ed. New York, NY: Oxford University Press.

Ji, Yu, Michael A. Garland, Bo Sun, Shuwen Zhang, Kurt Reynolds, Moira McMahon, Ratheya Rajakumar, et al. 2020. "Cellular and Developmental Basis of Orofacial Clefts." *Birth Defects Research* 112 (19): 1558–87. https://doi.org/10.1002/bdr2.1768.

Jiang, Rulang, Jeffrey O. Bush, and Andrew C. Lidral. 2006. "Development of the Upper Lip: Morphogenetic and Molecular Mechanisms." *Developmental Dynamics: An Official Publication of the American Association of Anatomists* 235 (5): 1152–66. https://doi.org/10.1002/dvdy.20646.

Johnson, J. M., G. Moonis, G. E. Green, R. Carmody, and H. N. Burbank. 2011. "Syndromes of the First and Second Branchial Arches, Part 1: Embryology and Characteristic Defects." *AJNR. American Journal of Neuroradiology* 32 (1): 14–19. https://doi.org/10.3174/ajnr.a2072.

Krauss, Robert S., and Mingi Hong. 2016. "Gene-Environment Interactions and the Etiology of Birth Defects." In *Current Topics in Developmental Biology*, 569–80. Elsevier.

Leslie, Elizabeth J., Jenna C. Carlson, John R. Shaffer, Azeez Butali, Carmen J. Buxó, Eduardo E. Castilla, Kaare Christensen, et al. 2017. "Genome-Wide Meta-Analyses of Nonsyndromic Orofacial Clefts Identify Novel Associations between FOXE1 and All Orofacial Clefts, and TP63 and Cleft Lip with or without Cleft Palate." *Human Genetics* 136 (3): 275–86. https://doi.org/10.1007/s00439-016-1754-7.

Leslie, Elizabeth J., and Mary L. Marazita. 2013. "Genetics of Cleft Lip and Cleft Palate: AMERICAN JOURNAL OF MEDICAL GENETICS PART C (SEMINARS IN MEDICAL GENETICS)." *American Journal of Medical Genetics. Part C, Seminars in Medical Genetics* 163 (4): 246–58. https://doi.org/10.1002/ajmg.c.31381.

Lidral, Andrew C., Lina M. Moreno, and Steven A. Bullard. 2008. "Genetic Factors and Orofacial Clefting." *Seminars in Orthodontics* 14 (2): 103–14. https://doi.org/10.1053/j.sodo.2008.02.002.

Mao, Jeremy J., and Hyun-Duck Nah. 2004. "Growth and Development: Hereditary and Mechanical Modulations." *American Journal of Orthodontics and Dentofacial Orthopedics: Official Publication of the American Association of Orthodontists, Its Constituent Societies, and the American Board of Orthodontics* 125 (6): 676–89. https://doi.org/10.1016/j.ajodo.2003.08.024.

Martinelli, Marcella, Annalisa Palmieri, Francesco Carinci and Luca Scapoli. 2020. "Non-Syndromic Cleft Palate: An Overview on Human Genetic and Environmental Risk Factors." *Frontiers in Cell and Developmental Biology* 8. https://doi.org/10.3389/fcell.2020.592271.

Nanci, A. 2013. *Ten cate, histologia oral*. 8th ed. Rio de Janeiro: Elsevier.

Nie, X., K. Luukko, and P. Kettunen. 2006. "FGF Signalling in Craniofacial Development and Developmental Disorders." *Oral Diseases* 12 (2): 102–11. https://doi.org/10.1111/j.1601-0825.2005.01176.x.

Online Mendelian Inheritance in Man, OMIM®. McKusick-Nathans Institute of Genetic Medicine, Johns Hopkins University (Baltimore, MD), (02 Dec 2022). World Wide Web URL: https://omim.org./

Ornoy, Asher. 2020. "Craniofacial Malformations and Their Association with Brain Development: The Importance of a Multidisciplinary Approach for Treatment." *Odontology* 108 (1): 1–15. https://doi.org/10.1007/s10266-019-00433-7.

Passos-Bueno, Maria Rita, Camila C. Ornelas, and Roberto D. Fanganiello. 2009. "Syndromes of the First and Second Pharyngeal Arches: A Review." *American Journal of Medical Genetics. Part A* 149A (8): 1853–59. https://doi.org/10.1002/ajmg.a.32950.

Rahimov, Fedik, Astanand Jugessur and Jeffrey C. Murray. 2012. "Genetics of Nonsyndromic Orofacial Clefts." *The Cleft Palate-Craniofacial Journal: Official Publication of the American Cleft Palate-Craniofacial Association* 49 (1): 73–91. https://doi.org/10.1597/10-178.

Reynolds, Kurt, Shuwen Zhang, Bo Sun, Michael A. Garland, Yu Ji and Chengji J. Zhou. 2020. "Genetics and Signaling Mechanisms of Orofacial Clefts." *Birth Defects Research* 112 (19): 1588–1634. https://doi.org/10.1002/bdr2.1754.

Roth, Daniela Marta, Francy Bayona, Pranidhi Baddam and Daniel Graf. 2021. "Craniofacial Development: Neural Crest in Molecular Embryology." *Head and Neck Pathology* 15 (1): 1–15. https://doi.org/10.1007/s12105-021-01301-z.

Setó-Salvia, Núria and Philip Stanier. 2014. "Genetics of Cleft Lip and/or Cleft Palate: Association with Other Common Anomalies." *European Journal of Medical Genetics* 57 (8): 381–93. https://doi.org/10.1016/j.ejmg.2014.04.003.

Shanske, Alan L. 2010. "Introductory Comments on Special Section-New Developments in Craniofacial Biology: Putting on a Happy Face." *American Journal of Medical Genetics. Part A* 152A (12): 2943–46. https://doi.org/10.1002/ajmg.a.33614.

Szabo-Rogers, Heather L., Lucy E. Smithers, Wardati Yakob and Karen J. Liu. 2010. "New Directions in Craniofacial Morphogenesis." *Developmental Biology* 341 (1): 84–94. https://doi.org/10.1016/j.ydbio.2009.11.021.

Tettamanti L, Avantaggiato A, Nardone M, Palmieri A, Tagliabue A. 2017. "New Insights in Orofacial Cleft: Epidemiological and Genetic Studies on Italian Samples." *Oral & Implantology* 10 (1): 11. https://doi.org/10.11138/orl/2017.10.1.011.

Twigg, Stephen R. F., and Andrew O. M. Wilkie. 2015. "New Insights into Craniofacial Malformations." *Human Molecular Genetics* 24 (R1): R50–59. https://doi.org/10.1093/hmg/ddv228.

Wieczorek, D. 2013. "Human Facial Dysostoses: Human Facial Dysostoses." *Clinical Genetics* 83 (6): 499–510. https://doi.org/10.1111/cge.12123.

Wilkie, Andrew O. M., and Gillian M. Morriss-Kay. 2001. "Genetics of Craniofacial Development and Malformation." *Nature Reviews. Genetics* 2 (6): 458–68. https://doi.org/10.1038/35076601.

Wójcicki, Piotr, Maciej Koźlik and Karolina Wójcicka. 2016. "Genetic Factors in Selected Complex Congenital Malformations with Cleft Defect." *Advances in Clinical and Experimental Medicine: Official Organ Wroclaw Medical University* 25 (5): 977–87. https://doi.org/10.17219/acem/61911.

Worley, Mitchell L., Krishna G. Patel, and Lauren A. Kilpatrick. 2018. "Cleft Lip and Palate." *Clinics in Perinatology* 45 (4): 661–78. https://doi.org/10.1016/j.clp.2018.07.006.

CHAPTER EIGHTEEN

CRANIOFACIAL DISORDERS ASSOCIATED WITH RARE FACIAL CLEFTS

Craniofacial Development

The skull and face develop from an orchestrated three-dimensional morphogenetic complex that involves several specific genes controlling a coordinated process of proliferation and cellular differentiation of embryological tissues. Craniofacial development is initiated by a dynamic temporospatial process that is highly susceptible to dysregulation and can result in congenital anomalies as well as facial clefts and craniofacial syndromes (Francis-West, Robson and Evans, 2003; Hennekam, Allanson and Krantz, 2010; Twigg and Wilkie, 2015; Roth et al. 2021).

Three successive stages characterize prenatal development. The first two, when combined, constitute the embryonic stage and the third is the foetal stage. The first phase begins at fertilization and comprises the first four weeks of development. This phase involves cell proliferation and migration, with some differentiation of cell populations. The second phase comprises the next four weeks of development and is characterized predominantly by the differentiation of all major internal and external structures (morphogenesis), called the embryonic stage. From the end of the second stage until parturition, further development is predominantly a matter of growth and maturation, and the embryo is called a foetus (Nanci 2013).

Early in morphogenesis, the skull and face develop through complex events mediated by cells derived from the neural crest, endoderm, mesoderm and ectoderm. Neural crest cells are multipotent and contribute mainly to forming facial tissues, bones, cartilage, and connective tissues (Caruso, Harris and Padwa, 2003; Mork and Crump, 2015; Graf et al., 2016).

In the embryo's dorsal ectoderm, neural crest cells are derived and migrate laterally to the neural tube. In the frontonasal process, these cells migrate to the cephalic region and contribute to developing the pharyngeal arches. The first and second arches are involved in forming the facial structures and are responsible for forming the maxillary and mandibular processes (Graf et al., 2016; Terrazas et al., 2017).

The frontonasal process develops in the ventrolateral region of the forebrain and is related to the formation of the frontal bone, nasal bridge, upper lip, philtrum and primary palate. Nasal placodes are derived from the frontonasal process and give rise to the medial and lateral nasal processes. The median nasal prominence expands until its fusion occurs, which determines the midline of the face and later contributes to the formation of the premaxilla, the philtrum, the columella, the tip and the cartilaginous septum of the nose. The lateral nasal processes give rise to the lateral portions of the nose (or alae nasi) (Caruso, Harris and Padwa, 2003; Som and Naidich, 2013; Cordero et al., 2011).

The maxillary processes, derived from the first pharyngeal arch, develop toward the midline and will form the maxilla, upper lip, central incisors, primary palate and zygoma. The mandibular processes, derived from the second pharyngeal arch, will fuse to form the mandible and the lower lip, formed by ectomensenchymal cells derived from this process (Caruso, Harris and Padwa, 2003).

The secondary palate develops from maxillary prominence, which the lateral palatine process projects medially in the form of palatine placodes that reach a horizontal position and fuse with the primary palate in the palatal midline. The incisive foramen marks the fuses between primary and secondary shelves, and posteriorly, the secondary palate formation is complete with fused palatal shelves and nasal septum (Nanci, 2013; Magreni and May 2015).

The upper portion and the middle face are derivated from the frontonasal process represented by the midline, frontal bone, nasal bridge and nasal tip. Their structures are derived from the maxillary process represented by the maxilla, zygoma, and lateral structures of the nose, and the lower region of the face is represented by the mandible and lower lip (Som and Naidich, 2013; Farlie et al. 2016).

The craniofacial development is determined by a complete migration of neural crest cells and by several signalling pathways, as well as BMP (bone morphogenetic proteins), WNT (wingless-related proteins), SHH (sonic hedgehog) and FGF (fibroblast growth factors), related to tissue differentiation and facial growth. Alterations in these signalling pathways can lead to several congenital anomalies in structures derived from the frontonasal process, resulting in facial clefts that can affect the frontal region, eyes, ears, nose, middle third of face, lip and palate (Szabo-Rogers et al. 2008; Sperber, Sperber; Guttmann, 2010; Marazita, 2012; Farlie et al. 2016; Graf et al. 2016).

The cleft lip and palate represent the most common craniofacial anomaly with complex aetiology, including genetic and environmental factors. They present variable forms and can affect only the lip, lip and palate or only the palate with involvement of uni or bilateral soft tissue and hard tissue structures (Tolarová and Cervenka, 1998; Mossey et al., 2009; Freitas et al., 2012; Marazita, 2012).

The other facial clefts are rare and represented by midline clefts, lateral clefts, oblique clefts and mandibular clefts. Each rare cleft described in the Tessier Classification has a distinct description for soft tissue and bone tissue, with a variable spectrum of severity (Tessier, 1976; Caruso, Harris and Padwa, 2003; Nanci, 2013; Winters, 2016).

References

Caruso, P. A., Harris, G. J., and Padwa, B. L. 2003. "CT imaging of craniofacial malformations." *Neuroimaging Clinics of North America* 13 (3): 541-572. https://doi.org/10.1016/s1052-5149(03)00061-3.

Cordero, D. R., Brugmann, S., Chu, Y., Bajpai, R., Jame, M., and Helms, J. A. 2011. "Cranial neural crest cells on the move: their roles in craniofacial development." American *Journal of Medical Genetics Part A* 155A (2): 270-279. https://doi.org/10.1002/ajmg.a.33702.

Farlie, P. G., Baker, N. L., Yap, P., and Tan, T. Y. 2016. "Frontonasal Dysplasia: Towards an Understanding of Molecular and Developmental Aetiology." *Molecular Syndromology* 7 (6): 312-332. https://doi.org/10.1159/000450533.

Francis-West, P. H., Robson, L., and Evans, D. J. 2003. "Craniofacial development: the tissue and molecular interactions that control development of the head." *Adv Anat Embryol Cell Biol*, 169, III-VI, 1-138. https://doi.org/10.1007/978-3-642-55570-1

Graf, D., Malik, Z., Hayano, S., and Mishina, Y. 2016. "Common mechanisms in development and disease: BMP signalling in craniofacial development." *Cytokine Growth Factor Rev*, 27, 129-139. https://doi.org/10.1016/j.cytogfr.2015.11.004.

Hennekam, R. C. M., Allanson, J. E., and Krantz, I. D. 2010. *Gorlin's Syndromes of Head and Neck.* New York: Oxford University Press.

Magreni, A., and May, J. G. 2015. “Embryology of the oral structures.” *Operative Techniques in Otolaryngology-Head and Neck Surgery*, 26(3), 110-114. https://doi.org/10.1016/j.otot.2015.06.002.

Marazita, M. L. 2012. The evolution of human genetic studies of cleft lip and cleft palate. *Annu Rev Genomics Hum Genet*, 13, 263-283. https://doi.org/10.1146/annurev-genom-090711-163729.

Mork, L., and Crump, G. 2015. “Zebrafish Craniofacial Development: A Window into Early Patterning.” *Curr Top Dev Biol*, 115, 235-269. https://doi.org/10.1016/bs.ctdb.2015.07.001.

Mossey, P. A., Little, J., Munger, R. G., Dixon, M. J., & Shaw, W. C. (2009). Cleft lip and palate. Lancet, 374(9703), 1773-1785. https://doi.org/10.1016/S0140-6736(09)60695-4

Nanci, A. (2013). *Ten cate, histologia oral*. 8th ed. Rio de Janeiro: Elsevier.

Roth, D. M., Bayona, F., Baddam, P., & Graf, D. (2021). Craniofacial Development: Neural Crest in Molecular Embryology. Head Neck Pathol, 15(1), 1-15. https://doi.org/10.1007/s12105-021-01301-z.

Som, P. M., & Naidich, T. P. (2013). Illustrated review of the embryology and development of the facial region, part 1: Early face and lateral nasal cavities. AJNR Am J Neuroradiol, 34(12), 2233-2240. https://doi.org/10.3174/ajnr.A3415.

Sperber, G. H., Sperber, S. M., & Guttmann, G. D. (2010). *Craniofacial embryogenetics and development*. 2nd ed. Shelton: PHPH-USA.

Szabo-Rogers, H. L., Geetha-Loganathan, P., Nimmagadda, S., Fu, K. K., & Richman, J. M. (2008). “FGF signals from the nasal pit are necessary for normal facial morphogenesis.” *Dev Biol*, 318(2), 289-302. https://doi.org/ 10.1016/j.ydbio.2008.03.027.

Terrazas, K., Dixon, J., Trainor, P. A., & Dixon, M. J. (2017). “Rare syndromes of the head and face: mandibulofacial and acrofacial dysostoses.” *Wiley Interdiscip Rev Dev Biol*, 6(3), 10.1002/wdev.263. https://doi.org/doi: 10.1002/wdev.263.

Tolarová, M. M., & Cervenka, J. (1998). "Classification and birth prevalence of orofacial clefts." *American Journal of Medical Genetics*, 75(2), 126-137.

Twigg, S. R., & Wilkie, A. O. (2015). "New insights into craniofacial malformations." *Human Molecular Genetics*, 24(R1), R50-R59. https://doi.org/10.1093/hmg/ddv228

Conditions with Rare Facial Clefts

Frontonasal Dysplasia

Frontonasal dysplasia (FND; OMIM 136760), also called median cleft syndrome and frontonasal malformation, is a condition characterized by the association of two or more of the following clinical findings: ocular hypertelorism, wide and broad nasal root, median cleft (affecting the nose only or the nose and upper lip), unilateral or bilateral nasal alae cleft, absence of nose tip formation, anterior cranium bifidum, and widow's peak (Sedano et al. 1970; Sedano and Gorlin 1988). It is considered a very heterogeneous group that includes the isolated and the syndromic form when associated with multiple anomalies, in which different associations constitute diverse and rare clinical conditions (Guion-Almeida et al. 1996; Wu, Vargevik and Slavotinek 2007; Umair et al. 2018).

The term "median cleft syndrome" was used by De Myer (1967) to describe this combination of anomalies. Later, the term "frontonasal dysplasia" was proposed by Sedano et al. (1970). After that, the term "frontonasal malformation" started to be used, with the justification that the combination of anomalies observed results from an alteration in the same developmental field (Sedano and Gorlin, 1988). Currently, it is known that this combination of clinical findings is a result of abnormal development of the frontonasal process, which is very important for proper face development and formation, starting at the fourth gestational week (Farlie et al. 2016; Lehalle et al. 2017).

Most cases of isolated FND are sporadic, and few cases of familial recurrence have been reported (Guion-Almeida et al. 1996). Regarding syndromic frontonasal dysplasia, some familial cases have been reported indicating autosomal dominant, autosomal recessive, and X-chromosome-linked inheritance models (Guion-Almeida et al. 1996; Wu, Vargevik, and Slavotinek, 2007; Lehalle et al. 2017). Pathogenic variants in EFNB1 (craniofrontonasal syndrome; OMIM 304110), ALX1 (FND type 3; OMIM 613456), ALX3 (FND type 1, frontorhiny; OMIM 136760) and ALX4 (FND type 2; OMIM 613451), ZSWIM6 (acromelic frontonasal dysostosis; OMIM 603671) and SPECC1L (Teebi hypertelorism syndrome; OMIM 145420) result in different conditions in which FND is part of the phenotype (Farlie et al. 2016; Lehalle et al. 2017; Umair et al. 2018). In addition to gene variations, environmental influences also appear to contribute to the occurrence of DFN (Twigg et al., 2009; Farlie et al., 2016). Some interesting examples of syndromic conditions with FND, unknown aetiology and rare clefts are Pai syndrome, oculoauriculofrontonasal syndrome and Sakoda complex.

Regarding rare clefts, the most common clefts in FND are the facial and cranial midline clefts (Tessier cleft numbers 0 and 14), observed with clinical variability and in several conditions, including isolated and syndromic FND. Besides that, alar clefts are also part of the phenotypic spectrum of FND, Tessier cleft number 2, and its craniofacial extension (Tessier number 12), being the most common (Sedano and Gorlin, 1988; Wu, Vargevik, and Slavotinek, 2007).

References

DeMyer, W. 1967. "The Median Cleft Face Syndrome. Differential Diagnosis of Cranium Bifidum Occultum, Hypertelorism and Median Cleft Nose, Lip and Palate". *Neurology* 17 (10): 961–71. https://doi.org/10.1212/wnl.17.10.961.

Farlie, Peter G., Naomi L. Baker, Patrick Yap and Tiong Y. Tan. 2016. "Frontonasal Dysplasia: Towards an Understanding of Molecular and Developmental Aetiology". *Molecular Syndromology* 7 (6): 312–21. https://doi.org/10.1159/000450533.

Guion-Almeida, M. L., A. Richieri-Costa, D. Saavedra, and M. M. Cohen Jr. 1996. "Frontonasal Dysplasia: Analysis of 21 Cases and Literature Review". *International Journal of Oral and Maxillofacial Surgery* 25 (2): 91–97. https://doi.org/10.1016/s0901-5027(96)80048-8.

Lehalle, Daphné, Umut Altunoglu, Ange-Line Bruel, Eric Arnaud, Patricia Blanchet, Jong-Woo Choi, Julie Désir, Esra Kiliç, Damien Lederer, Lucile Pinson, Christel Thauvin-Robinet, Amihood Singer, Julien Thevenon, Patrick Callier, Hulya Kayserili and Laurence Faivre. 2017. "Clinical Delineation of a Subtype of Frontonasal Dysplasia with Creased Nasal Ridge and Upper Limb Anomalies: Report of Six Unrelated Patients". *American Journal of Medical Genetics. Part A* 173 (12): 3136–42. https://doi.org/10.1002/ajmg.a.38490.

Sedano, Heddie O., M. Michael Cohen Jr, Jan Jirasek and Robert J. Gorlin. 1970. "Frontonasal Dysplasia". *The Journal of Pediatrics* 76 (6): 906–13. https://doi.org/10.1016/s0022-3476(70)80374-2.

Sedano, H. O., and R. J. Gorlin. 1988. "Frontonasal Malformation as a Field Defect and in Syndromic Associations". *Oral Surgery, Oral Medicine, and Oral Pathology* 65 (6): 704–10. https://doi.org/10.1016/0030-4220(88)90014-x.

Twigg, Stephen R. F., Sarah L. Versnel, Gudrun Nürnberg, Melissa M. Lees, Meenakshi Bhat, Peter Hammond, Raoul C. M. Hennekam, A. Jeannette M. Hoogeboom, Jane A. Hurst, David Johnson, Alexis A. Robinson, Peter J. Scambler, Dianne Gerrelli, Peter Nürnberg, Irene M. J. Mathijssen, and Andrew O. M. Wilkie. "Frontorhiny, a Distinctive Presentation of Frontonasal Dysplasia Caused by Recessive Mutations in the ALX3 Homeobox Gene". *The American Journal of Human Genetics* 84 (5): 698–705. https://doi.org/10.1016/j.ajhg.2009.04.009.

Umair, Muhammad, Farooq Ahmad, Muhammad Bilal and Muhammad Arshad. 2018. "Frontonasal dysplasia: a review". *Journal of Biochemical and Clinical Genetics*, 66–76. https://doi.org/10.24911/jbcgenetics/183-1530765389.

Wu, E., K. Vargevik, and A. M. Slavotinek. 2007. "Subtypes of Frontonasal Dysplasia Are Useful in Determining Clinical Prognosis". *American Journal of Medical Genetics. Part A* 143A (24): 3069–78. https://doi.org/10.1002/ajmg.a.31963.

Pai syndrome

Pai syndrome (OMIM 155145) is a rare condition characterized by median cleft, midline facial polyps, and pericallosal lipoma (Pai, Levkoff and Leithiser 1987; Guion-Almeida et al. 2007).

The median cleft is a frequent but variable finding. Most cases present a median cleft of the upper lip (Tessier cleft number 0) and duplicated maxillary frenulum (Lederer et al. 2012). However, there are severely affected cases that also present the craniofacial extension of the median cleft (Tessier cleft number 14), resulting in cranium bifidum occultum, severe ocular hypertelorism, and bifid nose (Guion-Almeida et al. 2007). Besides midline clefts (Tessier cleft numbers 0–14), other rare craniofacial clefts have been reported, including Tessier number 1 and number 3 clefts (Guion-Almeida et al. 2007).

Facial polyps can be unique or multiple, usually located in the facial midline. The most common are nasal polyps, arising from the nostrils or nasal dorsum (Castori et al. 2007). Although facial polyps are considered a hallmark of Pai syndrome, this clinical feature has been described in other conditions, including oculoauriculofrontonasal syndrome (OAFNS; OMIM 601452), Sakoda Complex (OMIM 610871), and encephalocraniocutaneous lipomatosis (ECCL; OMIM 613001) (Lehalle et al. 2022).

Additional frequent features of this syndrome include a wide spectrum of ocular anomalies, mainly epibulbar dermoids/lipodermoids and ocular hypertelorism (Guion-Almeida et al. 2007; Lederer et al. 2012; Li and Galvin 2017; Tormey, Cace and Boyle 2017; Morice et al. 2019). The association of ocular hypertelorism and median cleft characterizes frontonasal dysplasia (Sedano and Gorlin 1988), reported in some individuals with Pai syndrome (Guion-Almeida et al. 2007; Morice et al. 2019). Atypical additional findings reported include ear anomalies, preauricular tags, congenital heart anomalies, hypospadias, inguinal hernia, and vertebral malformations (Pai et al., 1987; Abdelmaaboud and Nimeri, 2012; Lederer et al., 2012; Li and Galvin 2017; Huckstadt et al. 2018; Morice et al. 2019; Olivero et al. 2020).

Nowadays, four diagnostic criteria are proposed. The first was proposed by Pai et al. (1987) and consisted of the triad of (1) median cleft lip, (2) midline skin polyps, and (3) pericallosal lipoma. Castori et al. (2007) proposed a clinical diagnosis based on the presence of at least two criteria: one or more hamartomatous nasal polyp(s) plus a midline facial cleft and/or mid-anterior alveolar process congenital polyp. Lederer et al. (2012) modified Castori's (2007) criteria to include pericallosal lipoma, resulting in a diagnostic criterion based on the presence of a congenital nasal polyp associated with one of the following: (1) median cleft lip, (2) mid-anterior alveolar process congenital polyp or (3) pericallosal lipoma. The literature review of 60 cases performed by Morice et al. (2019) evaluated the effectiveness of these criteria. Fewer than one-third of the cases met the criteria proposed by Pai et al. (1987); approximately 50% met the criteria by Castori et al. (2007); 80% met the criteria by Lederer et al. (2012). Based on these results, Morice et al. (2019) proposed an updated criterion: congenital nasal or mediofrontal skin mass and/or a mid-anterior alveolar mass polyp as mandatory criteria associated with at least one of the following criteria: (1) midline cleft lip and/or alveolar cleft; (2) pericallosal lipoma. 55 of 60 (91.7%) reported cases met the criteria proposed by Morice et al. (2019) for Pai syndrome.

The main differential diagnosis for Pai syndrome Is oculoauriculofrontonasal syndrome (OAFNS) (Lehalle et al. 2022). The case series reported by Lehalle et al. (2018) highlighted the presence of nasal polyps in 10 of 18 patients. Further, a literature review showed that nasal polyps have already been described in OAFNS (Lehalle et al. 2018). Additional features described in patients with Pai syndrome, including epibulbar dermoid, ear anomalies, preauricular tags and vertebral defects, reinforce the clinical overlap between these conditions (Abdelmaaboud and Nimeri, 2012; Li and Galvin, 2017; Huckstadt et al., 2018; Lehalle et al. 2018).

The aetiology of Pai syndrome remains unknown. Most cases are sporadic. Autosomal dominant inheritance has been suggested, but parental phenotype was unspecific and did not meet diagnostic criteria (Pai, Levkoff and Leithiser 1987; Rudnik-Schoneborn and Zerres 1994). Discordant monozygotic twins have been reported (Al-Mazrou et al. 2001). Cytogenetic investigation showed reciprocal translocation, 46,X,t(X;16)(q28;q11.2), in one case with median cleft lip and pedunculated skin polyps (Masuno et al. 1997). Recently, Lehalle et al. (2022) performed a molecular investigation on patients with Pai syndrome and overlapping conditions presenting facial polyps. Whole exome and genome sequencing identified only one *de novo* candidate variant in *TGFBRAP1*, a gene from the TGFβ pathway, absent in populational databases (gnomAD) and with an interesting bioinformatics score. Further molecular studies, considering the hypothesis of post-zygotic mosaicism, are necessary to elucidate this issue (Lehalle et al., 2022).

References

Abdelmaaboud, M., and N. Nimeri. 2012. "Pai Syndrome: First Reported Case in Qatar and Review of Literature of Previously Published Cases." *BMJ Case Reports*, no. 2012. https://doi.org/10.1136/bcr-02-2012-5940.

Al-Mazrou, Khalid A, Ammar Al-Rekabi, Ibrahim A Alorainy, Turki Al-Kharfi and Awad M Al-Serhani. 2001. "Pai Syndrome: A Report of a Case and Review of the Literature." *International Journal of Pediatric Otorhinolaryngology* 61, no. 2: 149–53. https://doi.org/10.1016/s0165-5876(01)00555-9.

Castori, Marco, Rosanna Rinaldi, Aurelia Bianchi, Aurelio Caponetti, Marcello Assumma and Paola Grammatico. 2007. "Pai Syndrome: First Patient with Agenesis of the Corpus Callosum and Literature Review." *Birth Defects Research Part A: Clinical and Molecular Teratology* 79, no. 10: 673–79. https://doi.org/10.1002/bdra.20392.

Guion-Almeida, Maria Leine, Cecília Mellado, Constanza Beltrán and Antonio Richieri-Costa. 2007. "Pai Syndrome: Report of Seven South American Patients." *American Journal of Medical Genetics Part A* 143A, no. 24: 3273–79. https://doi.org/10.1002/ajmg.a.31962.

Huckstadt, Victoria, María E. Heis Mendoza, Angélica Moresco and María G. Obregon. 2018. "Síndrome De Pai: Dos Nuevos Casos Con Manifestaciones Inusuales." *Archivos Argentinos de Pediatria* 116, no. 2: e336–e340. https://doi.org/10.5546/aap.2018.e336.

Lederer, Damien, Brian Wilson, Pierre Lefesvre, Vincent Vander Poorten, Nigel Kirkham, Dipayan Mitra, Christine Verellen-Dumoulin and Koenraad Devriendt. 2012. "Atypical Findings in Three Patients with Pai Syndrome and Literature Review." *American Journal of Medical Genetics Part A* 158A, no. 11: 2899–2904. https://doi.org/10.1002/ajmg.a.35592.

Lehalle, Daphné, Umut Altunoglu, Ange-Line Bruel, Mirna Assoum, Yannis Duffourd, Alice Masurel, Geneviève Baujat, Alice Goldenberg, Delphine Héron, Sarah Grotto, Sandrine Marlin, Audrey Putoux, Massimiliano Rossi, Pascale Saugier-Veber, Stéphane Triau, Christelle Cabrol, Myriam Vézain, Catherine Vincent-Delorme, Christel Thauvin-Robinet, Julien Thevenon, Pierre Vabres, Patrick Callier, Hulya Kayserili and Laurence Faivre. 2018. "The Oculoauriculofrontonasal Syndrome: Further Clinical Characterization and Additional Evidence Suggesting a Non-traditional Mode of Inheritance." *American Journal of Medical Genetics Part A*. https://doi.org/10.1002/ajmg.a.40662.

Lehalle, Daphné, Ange-Line Bruel, Antonio Vitobello, Anne-Sophie Denommé-Pichon, Yannis Duffourd, Mirna Assoum, Jeanne Amiel, Geneviève Baujat, Bettina Bessieres, Stefania Bigoni, Lydie Burglen, Guillaume Captier, Rodolphe Dard, Patrick Edery, Fernanda Fortunato, David Geneviève, Alice Goldenberg, Laurent Guibaud, Delphine Héron, Muriel Holder-Espinasse, Damien Lederer, Fermina Lopez Grondona, Sarah Grotto, Sandrine Marlin, Gwenael Nadeau, Arnaud Picard, Massimiliano Rossi, Joelle Roume, Damien Sanlaville, Pascale Saugier-Veber, Stéphane Triau, Maria Irene Valenzuela Palafoll, Clémence Vanlerberghe, Lionel Van Maldergem, Myriam Vezain, Catherine Vincent-Delorme, Einat Zivi, Julien Thevenon, Pierre Vabres, Christel Thauvin-Robinet, Patrick Callier and Laurence Faivre. 2022. "Toward Clinical and Molecular Dissection of Frontonasal Dysplasia with Facial Skin Polyps: From Pai Syndrome to Differential Diagnosis through a Series of 27 Patients." *American Journal of Medical Genetics Part A* 188, no. 7: 2036–47. https://doi.org/10.1002/ajmg.a.62739.

Li, Emily and Jennifer A. Galvin. 2017. "Ophthalmic Abnormalities of Pai Syndrome: A Case Report and Review of Literature." *Ophthalmic Genetics* 39, no. 2: 282–85. https://doi.org/10.1080/13816810.2017.1381979.

Masuno, M, K Imaizumi, Y Fukushima, Y Tanaka, T Ishii, M Nakamura and Y Kuroki. 1997. "Median Cleft of Upper Lip and Pedunculated Skin Masses Associated with De Novo Reciprocal Translocation 46,X,t(x;16)(q28;q11.2)." *Journal of Medical Genetics* 34, no. 11: 952–54. https://doi.org/10.1136/jmg.34.11.952.

Morice, A., E. Galliani, J. Amiel, M. Rachwalski, C. Neiva, C. Thauvin-Robinet, M.-P. Vazquez, A. Picard, and N. Kadlub. 2019. "Diagnostic Criteria in Pai Syndrome: Results of a Case Series and a Literature Review." *International Journal of Oral and Maxillofacial Surgery* 48, no. 3: 283–90. https://doi.org/10.1016/j.ijom.2018.08.010.

Olivero, Francesca, Thomas Foiadelli, Sabino Luzzi, Gian Luigi Marseglia and Salvatore Savasta. 2020. "Pai Syndrome: A Review." *Child's Nervous System* 36, no. 11: 2635–40. https://doi.org/10.1007/s00381-020-04788-z.

Online Mendelian Inheritance in Man, OMIM®. McKusick-Nathans Institute of Genetic Medicine, Johns Hopkins University (Baltimore, MD), (02 Dec 2022). World Wide Web URL: https://omim.org/

Pai, G. S., Abner H. Levkoff, and Richard E. Leithiser. 1987. "Median Cleft of the Upper Lip Associated with Lipomas of the Central Nervous System and Cutaneous Polyps." Edited by James F. Reynolds. *American Journal of Medical Genetics* 26, no. 4: 921–24.

https://doi.org/10.1002/ajmg.1320260421.

Rudnik-Schoneborn, S and K Zerres. 1994. "A Further Patient with Pai Syndrome with Autosomal Dominant Inheritance?" *Journal of Medical Genetics* 31, no. 6: 497–98. https://doi.org/10.1136/jmg.31.6.497.

Sedano, Heddie O., and Robert J. Gorlin. 1988. "Frontonasal Malformation as a Field Defect and in Syndromic Associations." *Oral Surgery, Oral Medicine, Oral Pathology* 65, no. 6: 704–10. https://doi.org/10.1016/0030-4220(88)90014-x.

Tormey, Peter, Iva Bilic Cace and Michael A. Boyle. 2017. "Ocular Dermoid in Pai Syndrome: A Review." *European Journal of Medical Genetics* 60, no. 4: 217–19. https://doi.org/10.1016/j.ejmg.2017.01.008.

Sakoda Complex

Sakoda et al. (1979) described a distinct combination of congenital anomalies in a male patient who presented with a median cleft lip/palate, sphenoethmoidal encephalomeningocele and agenesis of the corpus callosum. Later, this combination was denominated in the Sakoda complex (OMIM 610871) due to the addition of new features such as ocular anomalies, neurodevelopmental disturbance, and epilepsy (Dempsey, Torres-Martinez and Walsh 2007). Currently, it is considered a clinical spectrum (Ehara et al. 1998) and has also been suggested to be within the spectrum of frontonasal dysplasia syndromes (Richieri-Costa and Guion-Almeida 2004).

The median cleft is a common finding, with most cases presenting upper lip involvement (Tessier cleft number 0) (Ehara et al. 1998). Although it has never been described, the craniofacial extension of the median cleft (Tessier cleft number 14) is difficult to be evaluated on physical examination, but ocular hypertelorism and bifid nose could be clinical clues to the presence of this extension, and some patients had these findings described in the literature (Ehara et al. 1998; Richieri-Costa and Guion-Almeida 2004).

Corpus callosum agenesis is one of the most common congenital cerebral anomalies and has already been described in isolated and syndromic cases, with over 200 different syndromes described so far (Das and Geetha, 2022). On the Sakoda spectrum, the agenesis of the corpus callosum has been described in most cases (Ehara et al. 1998; Richieri-Costa and Guion-Almeida 2004), although it is considered a cardinal feature, which could explain the high frequency.

The basal encephalomeningocele is characterized by a defect of the anterior cranial fossa, leading to the herniation of the meninges and brain. It is classified based on topography: transethmoidal, sphenoethmoidal, transsphenoidal, and frontosphenoidal or spheno-orbital (Ehara et al. 1998). This encephalocele has been identified as an isolated feature or associated with other anomalies. Syndromic cases were mainly described in the Sakoda complex and with frontonasal dysplasia. Although the sphenoethmoidal type is the best described, the trans-sphenoidal type has also been described within the Sakoda spectrum (Ehara et al. 1998; Richieri-Costa and Guion-Almeida 2004).

The ocular anomalies associated with the Sakoda spectrum are extremely variable. However, the most common is the 'morning glory' anomaly, defined as a large optic nerve and funnelled, which displays a conical excavation of the optic disc appearing dysplastic, resembling the flower with the same name (Ehara et al. 1998). Microphthalmia, colobomas, anophthalmia, microcorneas, cataracts, ocular proptosis and ptosis have also been described (Ehara et al. 1998; Richieri-Costa and Guion-Almeida 2004).

Lees et al. (1998) emphasized the importance of evaluating individuals with midline anomalies, including a median cleft and encephaloceles, for endocrinologic disturbances, such as diabetes insipidus and pituitary dysfunction.

Currently, no diagnostic criteria have been proposed. However, in the presence of a median cleft (Tessier cleft number 0), basal encephalomeningocele, the morning glory anomaly and/or agenesis of the corpus callosum, and the Sakoda spectrum should be considered a differential diagnosis.

The aetiology of this entity remains unknown, with most cases being sporadic. Guion-Almeida et al. (2012) described a female with Sakoda spectrum features and a partial 21q22.3 deletion, suggesting that genes within this region could account for the phenotype. Molecular investigation in other patients with Sakoda complex, focused on *TGIF*, *ALX3* and *ALX4* genes, also has been made, but no mutation was identified (Guion-Almeida et al. 2012).

References

Das, Joe M, Ragi Geetha. "Corpus Callosum Agenesis". 2022. In: *StatPearls*. Treasure Island (FL): StatPearls Publishing. https://www.ncbi.nlm.nih.gov/books/NBK540986/.

Dempsey, Melissa A., Wilfredo Torres-Martinez and Laurence E. Walsh. 2007."Two cases further delineating the Sakoda complex". *American Journal of Medical Genetics Part A* 143A, n.º 4: 370–76. https://doi.org/10.1002/ajmg.a.31582.

Ehara, Hiroaki, Akihiro Kurimasa, Kousaku Ohno and Kenzo Takeshita. 1998. "New Syndrome With the Sakoda Complex, Bilateral Anophthalmia and Cortical Dysgenesi". *Pediatric Neurology* 18, n.º 5: 445–51. https://doi.org/10.1016/s0887-8994(97)00231-2.

Guion-Almeida, Maria Leine, Antonio Richieri-Costa, Fernanda Sarquis Jehee, Maria Rita Santos Passos-Buenoande Roseli Maria Zechi-Ceide. 2012."Frontonasal dysplasia, callosal agenesis, basal encephalocele and eye anomalies syndrome with a partial 21q22.3 deletion". *American Journal of Medical Genetics Part A* 158A, n.º 7: 1676–79. https://doi.org/10.1002/ajmg.a.35351.

Lees, M. M., P. Hodgkins, W. Reardon, D. Taylor, R. Stanhope, B. Jones, R. Hayward, A. D. Hockley, M. Baraitser and R. M. Winter. 1998."Frontonasal dysplasia with optic disc anomalies and other midline craniofacial defects: a report of six cases". *Clinical Dysmorphology* 7, n.º 3: 157–62. https://doi.org/10.1097/00019605-199807000-00001.

Richieri-Costa, Antonio and Maria Leine Guion-Almeida. 2004."The Syndrome of Frontonasal Dysplasia, Callosal Agenesis, Basal Encephalocele and Eye Anomalies – Phenotypic and Aetiological Consideration". *International Journal of Medical Sciences* 1, n.º 1: 34–42. https://doi.org/10.7150/ijms.1.34.

Sakoda, Katsuaki, Susumu Ishikawa, Tohru Uozumi, Katsuhiro Hirakawa, Hideo Okazaki e Yasuo Harada. 1979. "Sphenoethmoidal meningoencephalocele associated with agenesis of corpus callosum and median cleft lip and palate". *Journal of Neurosurgery* 51, n.º 3: 397–401. https://doi.org/10.3171/jns.1979.51.3.0397.

Oculoauriculofrontonasal syndrome

The oculoauriculofrontonasal syndrome (OAFNS; OMIM 601452) is a rare condition characterized by the association of clinical features of frontonasal dysplasia and oculoauriculovertebral spectrum (Evans et al. 2013; Lehalle et al. 2018). Frontonasal dysplasia (FND) is described as the association of at least two of the following features: widow's peak, true ocular hypertelorism, broad or bifid nose, nasal cleft, absence of a nasal tip, median cleft, and anterior cranium bifidum (Sedano and Gorlin 1988). The oculoauriculovertebral spectrum (OAVS) is characterized by ear anomalies or preauricular tags and mandibular hypoplasia, although no minimum criteria are established, and clinical diagnostic criteria are variable (Rollnick et al. 1987; Barisic et al. 2014; Beleza-Meireles et al. 2014).

Considering the clinical overlap, rare craniofacial clefts commonly observed in DFN and OAVS have been described in the OAFNS, especially those affecting the craniofacial midline, nose, and mandible (Gupta, Gupta and Prashar 1968; Naidich et al. 1988; Toriello, Higgins and Mann 1995; Al-Gazali et al. 1996; Román Corona-Rivera et al. 2007; Gabbett et al. 2008; Adolphs et al. 2012; Evans et al. 2013; Tunc et al. 2017; Lehalle et al. 2018; Ito et al. 2019; Serigatto et al. 2023). The most frequently reported rare craniofacial clefts in OAFNS are Tessier cleft numbers 0–14, 2–12, and 7 (Evans et al. 2013). Further rare craniofacial clefts described in OAFNS include Tessier cleft numbers 1–13, 6, 8, and 10 (Naidich et al. 1988; Adolphs et al. 2012; Serigatto et al. 2023). Moreover, the mandibular cleft (Tessier cleft number 30) has already been described in OAFNS (Lehalle et al. 2018).

In summary, the main clinical features of OAFNS include ocular hypertelorism, a broad nose, mandibular hypoplasia, preauricular tags, microtia, and facial asymmetry (Gabbett et al. 2008; Lehalle et al. 2018). The diagnostic criteria proposed by Lehalle et al. (2018) consist of the presence of ocular hypertelorism, preauricular tags or microtia, and facial asymmetry, and the three mandatory findings, in addition to the most common features of DFN, such as a broad or cleft nose, and OAVS, such as epibulbar dermoid. Despite the similarities, the OAFNS has been considered a distinct condition, not just a subgroup within the FND or OAVS (Carey et al. 1996; Gabbett et al. 2008; Evans et al. 2013; Lehalle et al. 2018). An exclusive radiological finding that contributed to recognising OAFNS as a distinct condition was the ectopic nasal bone (Evans et al. 2013). The ectopic nasal bone is a bone structure that is observed in approximately 30% of individuals with OAFNS and presents clinical variability, ranging from dysplastic nasal bones to complete dysmorphic spoon-shaped bones or bone bridges that connect the nasal bones to the premaxilla (Evans et al. 2013; Serigatto et al. 2023). The frequencies of clinical findings and description of unique features, such as the ectopic nasal bone, reinforce the classification of OAFNS as a distinct condition (Evans et al. 2013; Lehalle et al. 2018). To date, over 60 individuals with OAFNS have been reported in the literature (Gabbett et al. 2008; Evans et al. 2013; Lehalle et al. 2018; Ito et al. 2019; Serigatto et al. 2023).

The main differential diagnosis for OAFNS includes FND, OAVS and Pai syndrome. The clinical overlap with Pai syndrome was reinforced due to facial polyps associated with ocular hypertelorism and midline cleft in individuals with OAFNS (Lehalle et al. 2018). Furthermore, several individuals with OAFNS presenting nasal polyps have been reported (Musarella and Young 1986; Al-Gazali et al. 1996; Casey et al. 1996; Román Corona-Rivera et al. 2007; Borumandi et al. 2015; Lehalle et al. 2018).

The aetiology of OAFNS remains unknown; most cases reported are sporadic. A recurrence in siblings was reported in one case, suggesting autosomal recessive inheritance (Golabi, Gonzales and Edwards 1983). However, segregation analysis excluded this hypothesis (Gabbett et al., 2008). Cytogenetics and molecular investigation, including whole genome sequencing, showed no results (Evans et al. 2013; Lehalle et al. 2018). These findings suggest non-traditional inheritance models for OAFNS, for example, mosaicism, epigenetic mechanism, or a non-genetic cause (Lehalle et al. 2018).

References

Adolphs, Nicolai, Eric Arnaud, Ernst-Johannes Haberl, Luitgard Graul-Neumann, Gül Schmidt, Horst Menneking and Bodo Hoffmeister. 2012. "The Oculo-Auriculo-Fronto-Nasal Syndrome (OAFNS) – Description of a Rare and Complex Craniofacial Deformity and Its Interdisciplinary Management before School Age." *Journal of Cranio-Maxillofacial Surgery* 40, no. 8: 668–74. https://doi.org/10.1016/j.jcms.2011.11.003.

Al-Gazali, L. I., A. H. Dawodu, M. Hamada, M. Bakir, and D. Bakalinová. 1996. "Severe Facial Clefting, Limbic Dermoid, Hypoplasia of the Corpus Callosum, and Multiple Skin Appendages: Severe Frontofacionasal 'Dysplasia' or Newly Recognised Syndrome?" *American Journal of Medical Genetics* 63, no. 2: 346–47. https://doi.org/10.1002/(sici)1096-8628(19960517)63:2<346::aid-ajmg4>3.0.co;2-r

Barisic, Ingeborg, Ljubica Odak, Maria Loane, Ester Garne, Diana Wellesley, Elisa Calzolari, Helen Dolk, Marie-Claude Addor, Larraitz Arriola, Jorieke Bergman, Sebastiano Bianca, Berenice Doray, Babak Khoshnood, Kari Klungsoyr, Bob McDonnell, Anna Pierini, Judith Rankin, Anke Rissmann,Catherine Rounding, Annette Queisser-Luft, Gioacchino Scarano & David Tucker. 2014. "Prevalence, Prenatal Diagnosis and Clinical Features of Oculo-Auriculo-Vertebral Spectrum: A Registry-Based Study in Europe." *European Journal of Human Genetics* 22, 8 (2014): 1026–33. https://doi.org/10.1038/ejhg.2013.287.

Beleza-Meireles, Ana, Jill Clayton-Smith, Jorge M Saraiva and May Tassabehji. 2014. "Oculo-Auriculo-Vertebral Spectrum: A Review of the Literature and Genetic Update." *Journal of Medical Genetics* 51, no. 10: 635–45. https://doi.org/ 10.1136/jmedgenet-2014-102476.

Borumandi, Farzad, Ambika Chadha, Emil Dediol and Vedran Uglešić. 2015. "A Diagnostic Conundrum: Ectopic Nasal Ossification, Submucosal Alveolar Cleft, Absent Posterior Atlantal Arch and Corpus Callosum Lipoma." *The Cleft Palate-Craniofacial Journal* 52, no. 6: 761–65. https://doi.org/10.1597/14-108.

Casey, Holly D., Stephen R. Braddock, Richard C. Haskins, John C. Carey, and Louis, Morales. 1996. "Frontonasal Malformation and the Oculoauriculovertebral Spectrum: The Oculoauriculofrontonasal Syndrome." *The Cleft Palate-Craniofacial Journal* 33, no. 6 (1996): 519–23.
https://doi.org/10.1597/1545-1569_1996_033_0519_fmatos_2.3.co_2.

Evans, Kelly N., Joseph S. Gruss, Paritosh C. Khanna, Michael L. Cunningham, Timothy C. Cox, and Anne V. Hing. 2013. "Oculoauriculofrontonasal Syndrome: Case Series Revealing New Bony Nasal Anomalies in an Old Syndrome." *American Journal of Medical Genetics* Part A 161, no. 6 (2013): 1345–53.
https://doi.org/10.1002/ajmg.a.35926.

Gabbett, Michael T., Stephen P. Robertson, Roland Broadbent, Salim Aftimos, Rani Sachdev and Marjan M. Nezarati. 2008. "Characterizing the Oculoauriculofrontonasal Syndrome." *Clinical Dysmorphology* 17, no. 2 (2008): 79–85. https://doi.org/10.1097/mcd.0b013e3282f449c8.

Golabi, M., M. C. Gonzales, and M. S. Edwards. 1983. "A new syndrome of oculoauriculovertebral dysplasia and midline craniofacial defect: the oculoauriculofrontonasal syndrome. Two new cases in sibs." *Birth Defects* 19, no. 5: 183-184.

Gupta, J S, S D Gupta and S K Prashar. 1968. "Oculo-Auricular Cranial Dysplasia." *British Journal of Ophthalmology* 52, no. 4: 346–47. https://doi.org/10.1136/bjo.52.4.346.

Ito, Riri, Masayuki Osawa, Yuhei Yamamoto, Naoki Murao, Toshihiko Hayashi, Taku Maeda, Kosuke Ishikawa, Akihiko Oyama and Emi Funayama. 2019. "Oculo-Auriculo-Fronto-Nasal Syndrome with Duane Retraction Syndrome and Dysplastic Bony Structure in the Midline of Nose." *Journal of Craniofacial Surgery* 30, no. 6. https://doi.org/10.1097/scs.0000000000005636.

Lehalle, Daphné, Umut Altunoglu, Ange-Line Bruel, Mirna Assoum, Yannis Duffourd, Alice Masurel, Geneviève Baujat, Alice Goldenberg, Delphine Héron, Sarah Grotto, Sandrine Marlin, Audrey Putoux, Massimiliano Rossi, Pascale Saugier-Veber, Stéphane Triau, Christelle Cabrol, Myriam Vézain, Catherine Vincent-Delorme, Christel Thauvin-Robinet, Julien Thevenon, Pierre Vabres, Patrick Callier, Hulya Kayserili and Laurence Faivre. 2018. "The Oculoauriculofrontonasal Syndrome: Further Clinical Characterization and Additional Evidence Suggesting a Non-traditional Mode of Inheritance." *American Journal of Medical Genetics Part A*, 176(12):2740-2750. https://doi.org/10.1002/ajmg.a.40662.

Musarella, Maria A., and Ian D. Young. 1986. "A Patient with Median Cleft Face Anomaly and Bilateral Goldenhar Anomaly." *American Journal of Medical Genetics* 25, no. S2: 135–41. https://doi.org/10.1002/ajmg.1320250617.

Naidich, Thomas P., Robin E. Osborn, Bruce Bauer and Michelle J. Naidich. 1988. "Median Cleft Face Syndrome: MR and CT Data from 11 Children." *Journal of Computer Assisted Tomography* 12, no. 1: 57–64. https://doi.org/10.1097/00004728-198801000-00011.

Online Mendelian Inheritance in Man, OMIM®. McKusick-Nathans Institute of Genetic Medicine, Johns Hopkins University (Baltimore, MD), (02 Dec 2022). World Wide Web URL: https://omim.org./

Rollnick, Beverly R., Celia I. Kaye, Konrad Nagatoshi, Walter Hauck and Alice O. Martin. 1987. "Oculoauriculovertebral Dysplasia and Variants: Phenotypic Characteristics of 294 Patients." *American Journal of Medical Genetics* 26, no. 2: 361–75. https://doi.org/10.1002/ajmg.1320260215.

Román Corona-Rivera, Jorge, Eloy López-Marure, Larissa Gómez-Ruíz, María del Carmen Abreu-Fernández, Claudia Quezada-López, Jesús Pérez-Molina and Laura Patricia Santibañez-Escobar. 2007. "Airway Anomalies in the Oculoauriculofrontonasal Syndrome." *Clinical Dysmorphology* 16, no. 1: 43–45. https://doi.org/10.1097/mcd.0b013e328010d402.

Sedano, Heddie O., and Robert J. Gorlin. 1988. “Frontonasal Malformation as a Field Defect and in Syndromic Associations.” *Oral Surgery, Oral Medicine, Oral Pathology* 65, no. 6: 704–10. https://doi.org/10.1016/0030-4220(88)90014-x.

Serigatto, Henrique R., Nancy M. Kokitsu-Nakata, Priscila P. Moura, Siulan Vendramini-Pittoli, Luiza A. Virmond, Adriano P. Peixoto, Cristiano Tonello, Luciano A. Brito, Maria R. Passos-Bueno, and Roseli M. Zechi-Ceide. “Complex Craniofacial Cleft and Accessory Maxilla in Oculoauriculofrontonasal Syndrome.” 2023. *Clinical Dysmorphology* 32, no.1: 21–24. https://doi.org/10.1097/mcd.0000000000000434.

Toriello, H. V., J. V. Higgins, and R. Mann. 1995. “Oculoauriculofrontonasal Syndrome: Report of Another Case and Review of Differential Diagnosis.” *Clinical Dysmorphology* 4, no. 4: 338–46. https://doi.org/10.1097/00019605-199510000-00010.

Tunc, Turan, Adem Polat, Bilal Altan, Abdul Kerim Yapici, Mehmet Saldir, Sabahattin Sari, Erkan Sari, Yalcin Bayram and Muhitdin Eski. 2017. “Oculoauriculofrontonasal Dysplasia Syndrome with Additional Clinical Features.” *The Cleft Palate-Craniofacial Journal* 54, no. 6: 749–53. https://doi.org/10.1597/15-078.

Facial dysostosis

Facial dysostosis represents a group genetically heterogeneous with craniofacial anomalies that affect structures derived from the first and second pharyngeal arches. Clinically, they present a combination of facial tissue deficiencies and facial hypoplasia, including maxilla and complex zygomatic hypoplasia, mandibular hypoplasia, ear anomalies (external and middle), and orofacial clefts may be present. This condition can be subdivided into acrofacial dysostosis when the craniofacial anomalies occur associated with limb anomalies, and mandibulofacial dysostosis when only craniofacial anomalies are present. Radiologically, it is possible to evaluate bone anomalies, including rare facial clefts (or Tessier clefts), in some of these conditions (Hennekam, Allanson, Krantz, 2010; Trainor and Andrews, 2013; Wieczorek, 2013).

References

Hennekam, Raoul, Judith E. Allanson, and Ian Krantz. 2010. *Gorlin's Syndromes of the Head and Neck*. 5th ed. New York, NY: Oxford University Press.

Trainor, P. A., and Andrews, B. T. 2013. "Facial dysostoses: etiology, pathogenesis and management." *American Journal of Medical Genetics Part C: Seminars in Medical Genetics*, vol. 163C, no. 4, pp. 283–294. https://doi.org/ 10.1002/ajmg.c.31375.

Wieczorek, D. 2013. "Human facial dysostoses." *Clinical Genetics*, vol. 83, no. 6, pp. 499-510. https://doi.org/10.1111/cge.12123.

Mandibulofacial dysostosis (MFD)

Treacher Collins syndrome (TCS)

The most common condition in the group of MFDs was initially recognized as a syndrome in 1900 by Treacher Collins and later classified as mandibulofacial dysostosis by Franceschetti and Klein in 1949. It has an incidence of 1:50,000 live births, with no preferences for gender; familial recurrence has been observed in 40% of cases and 60% result in spontaneous or *de novo* mutations (van Gijn, Tucker and Couborne 2012; Trainor and Andrews 2013; Aljerian and Gilardino, 2019).

It is a genetically heterogeneous condition with wide intra and interfamilial clinical variability. Until now, four genes related to this condition have been described in the literature. The *TCOF1* gene is related to TCS1 (OMIM 154500), and this represents most cases; the *POLR1D* gene is related to TCS2 (OMIM 613717), the *POLR1C* gene is related to TCS3 (OMIM 248390) and the *POLR1B* gene is related to TCS4 (OMIM 618939) (Marszałek-Kruk et al. 2021)

Clinically, it presents bilateral hypoplasia of the facial bones, particularly affecting the mandible (78%) and zygomatic complex (81%). Its effects may present in the following ways: down slanting palpebral fissures, coloboma in the lower eyelid and cleft palate, auricular anomalies and an absence of the auditory canal and hearing loss. Other less frequent clinical signs include microcephaly, developmental delay, and intellectual disability (Dixon, Trainor and Dixon 2007; Dauwerse et al. 2011; Trainor 2010; Schlump et al. 2012).

Tessier's clefts are also observed in the clinical characteristics of TCS, both in the soft and bone tissue. The most frequent is cleft number 6 (maxillozygomatic), which presents a cleft between the maxilla and the zygomatic bone in the infraorbital region, and in the soft tissue, it presents a furrow in the cheek. Cleft number 7 (temporozygomatic), which can present a cleft in the zygomatic arch or a complete absence of the arch, is associated with condyle anomalies, coronoid process anomalies and in the soft tissue, it presents macrostomia. Cleft number 8 (frontozygomatic), which presents a cleft in the lateral margin of the orbit and the soft tissue, shows a defect in the external palpebral commissure (Tessier, 1976; Weinzweig 2010; Cobb et al. 2014; Franchi et al. 2015).

References

Aljerian, A., and Gilardino, M.S. 2019. "Treacher Collins Syndrome." Clinical Plastic Surgery, vol. 46, no. 2, pp. 197-205. https://doi.org/10.1016/j.cps.2018.11.005.

Cobb, A. R., Green, B., Gill, D., Ayliffe, P., Lloyd, T. W., Bulstrode, N., and Dunaway, D. J. 2014. "The surgical management of Treacher Collins syndrome." *British Journal of Oral and Maxillofacial Surgery*, vol. 52, no. 7, pp. 581-589. https://doi.org/10.1016/j.bjoms.2014.02.007.

Dauwerse, J. G., Dixon, J., Seland, S., Ruivenkamp, C. A., van Haeringen, A., Hoefsloot, L. H. Dorien, J. P., Clement-de Boers, A., Daumer-Haas, C., Maiwald, R., Zweier, C., Kerr, B., Cobo, A. M., Toral, J. F., Hoogeboom, A. J. M., Dietmar R Lohmann, D. R., Ute Hehr, U., Dixon, M. J., Breuning, M. H., Dagmar Wieczorek. D. 2011. "Mutations in genes encoding subunits of RNA polymerases I and III cause Treacher Collins syndrome." *Nature Genetics*, vol. 43, no. 1, pp. 20-22. https://doi.org/10.1038/ng.724.

Dixon, J., Trainor, P., and Dixon, M. J. 2007. "Treacher Collins syndrome." *Orthodontics and Craniofacial Research*, vol. 10, no. 2, pp. 88-95. https://doi.org/ 10.1111/j.1601-6343.2007.00388.x.

Franchi, G., Kadlub, N., Diner, P. A., Bandini, M., Vazquez, M. P., and Picard, A. 2015. "Orbital soft tissue surgery for patients with Treacher Collins or Nager syndrome: A new surgical approach with early correction of soft tissue: prospective study." *British Journal of Oral and Maxillofacial Surgery*, vol. 53, no. 5, pp. 421-425. https://doi.org/ 10.1016/j.bjoms.2015.02.004.

Hennekam, Raoul, Judith E. Allanson, and Ian Krantz. 2010. *Gorlin's Syndromes of the Head and Neck*. 5th ed. New York, NY: Oxford University Press.

Kadakia, S., Helman, S. N., Badhey, A. K., Saman, M., and Ducic, Y. 2014. "Treacher Collins Syndrome: The genetics of a craniofacial disease." *International Journal of Pediatric Otorhinolaryngology*, vol. 78, no. 6, pp. 893-898. https://doi.org/ 10.1016/j.ijporl.2014.03.006.

Lehalle, D., Wieczorek, D., Zechi-Ceide, RM., Passos-Bueno, MR., Lyonnet, S., Amiel, J., and Gordon, CT. 2015. "A review of craniofacial disorders caused by spliceosomal defects." *Clinical Genetics*, vol. 88, no. 5, pp. 405-415. https://doi.org/10.1111/cge.12596.

Marszałek-Kruk, B. A., Wójcicki, P., Dowgierd, K., & Śmigiel, R. 2021. "Treacher Collins Syndrome: Genetics, Clinical Features and Management." *Genes*, 12(9), 1392.

https://doi.org/10.3390/genes12091392.
Online Mendelian Inheritance in Man, OMIM®. McKusick-Nathans Institute of Genetic Medicine, Johns Hopkins University (Baltimore, MD), (02 Dec 2022). World Wide Web URL: https://omim.org/.
Plomp, R. G., et al. (2016). "Treacher Collins Syndrome: A Systematic Review of Evidence-Based Treatment and Recommendations." *Plast Reconstr Surg*, 137(1), 191-204. https://doi.org/ 10.1097/PRS.0000000000001896.
Schlump, Stein, A., Ute Hehr, U., Karen, T., Möller-Hartmann, C., Elcioglu, N. H., Bogdanova, N., Hartmut Fritz Woike, H. F., Lohmann, D. R., Ursula Felderhoff-Mueser, U., Annette Linz, A., Wieczorek, D. 2012. "Treacher Collins syndrome: clinical implications for the paediatrician-a new mutation in a severely affected newborn and comparison with three further patients with the same mutation, and review of the literature." *Eur J Pediatr*, 171(11), 1611-1618. https://doi.org/10.1007/s00431-012-1776-7.
Tessier, P. 1976. "Anatomical classification facial, cranio-facial and latero-facial clefts." *J Maxillofac Surg*, 4(2), 69-92.
Trainor, P. A. 2010. "Craniofacial birth defects: the role of neural crest cells in the etiology and pathogenesis of Treacher Collins syndrome and the potential prevention." *Am J Med Genet A*, 152A(12), 2984-2994. https://doi.org/ 10.1002/ajmg.a.33454.
Trainor, P. A., and Andrews, B. T. 2013. "Facial dysostoses: etiology, pathogenesis and management." *American Journal of Medical Genetics Part C: Seminars in Medical Genetics*, vol. 163C, no. 4, pp. 283-294. https://doi.org/ 10.1002/ajmg.c.31375.
van Gijn, D. R., Tucker, A. S., & Cobourne, M. T. 2013. "Craniofacial development: current concepts in the molecular basis of Treacher Collins syndrome." Br J Oral Maxillofac Surg, 51(5), 384-388. https://doi.org/ 10.1016/j.bjoms.2012.09.008.
Weinzweig, J. 2010. *Plastic surgery secrets plus*. Elsevier Health Sciences.
Wieczorek, D. 2013. "Human facial dysostoses." *Clinical Genetics*, vol. 83, no. 6, pp. 499-510. https://doi.org/10.1111/cge.12123.

Mandibulofacial dysostosis Guion-Almeida type (MFDGA)

Mandibulofacial dysostosis Guion-Almeida type, as mandibulofacial dysostosis with microcephaly is called (OMIM 610536), was initially described by Guion-Almeida et al. (2006) in four Brazilian individuals (three males and one female). It is mainly characterized by weight and height deficit, micro trigonocephaly, hypoplasia of the zygomatic arch, micrognathia, cleft palate/Robin sequence, mandibulofacial dysostosis, small and prominent ears with helix, antihelix, tragus and lobe anomalies, preauricular appendage, a significant delay in neuropsychomotor development, a delay in speech acquisition and language delay. Later, Guion-Almeida et al. (2009) described two other cases with this condition, a male and his mother, with probable autosomal dominant inheritance. However, X-linked recessive inheritance cannot be excluded. The proband's mother presented, in addition to the characteristic facial clinical signs of the condition, mandibular and epibulbar dermoid asymmetry.

Wieczoreck et al. (2009) described three unrelated patients with microcephaly, microtia with a preauricular and facial appendage, choanal atresia and delay in neuropsychomotor development.

Lines et al. (2012) identified in molecular analysis a heterozygous pathogenic variant of the *EFTUD2* gene (17q21.31) in all 12 individuals studied and concluded that haploinsufficiency of the *EFTUD2* gene was responsible for mandibulofacial dysostosis Guion-Almeida type, including two cases described by Guion-Almeida and three cases described by Wieczoreck et al. (2009).

Currently, many studies have been carried out on individuals with MFDGA around the world. Another 108 cases have been documented, and it is the second best-known MFD (Huang et al. 2015; Dragoi et al. 2021).

In additional, Luquetti et al. (2013), expanding the phenotype, showed the presence of Tessier cleft number 7 (temporozygomatic) in computed tomography performed in individuals with MFDGA. In the radiological analysis, it was possible to observe complete zygomatic arch clefting in two cases and unilateral in one case, with severe bilateral maxillary hypoplasia in all the cases.

References

Dragoi V, Nedelea F, Gica N, Botezatu R, Peltecu G, Panaitescu AM. 2021. "Prenatal features of mandibulofacial dysostosis Guion-Almeida Type." *J Med Life*. Sep-Oct;14(5):722-725. https://doi.org10.25122/jml-2020-0082.

Guion-Almeida, M. L., Vendramini-Pitolli, S., Passos-Bueno, M. R., and Zechi-Ceide, R. M. 2009. "Mandibulofacial syndrome with growth and mental retardation, microcephaly, ear anomalies with skin tags and cleft palate in a mother and her son: autosomal dominant or X-linked syndrome?" *Am J Med Genet*, 149A(12), 2762-2764. https://doi.org/ 10.1002/ajmg.a.32816.

Guion-Almeida, M. L., Zechi-Ceide, R. M., Vendramini, S., and Tabith, A. J. 2006. "A new syndrome with growth and mental retarding, mandibulofacial dysostosis, microcephaly and cleft palate." *Clin Dysmorphol*, 15(3), 171-174. https://doi.org/ 10.1097/01.mcd.0000220603.09661.7e

Huang, L., Vanstone, M. R., Hartley, T., Osmond, M., Barrowman, N., Allanson, J., Baker, L. Tabib A Dabir, T. A., Katrina M Dipple, K. M., Dobyns W. B., Jane Estrella, J., Hanna Faghfoury, H., Favaro, F.P., Himanshu Goel, H., Pernille A Gregersen, P. A., Karen W Gripp, K. W., Art Grix, A., Guion-Almeida, M.L., Harr, M. H., Hudson, C., Hunter, A. W., Johnson, J., Joss, S. K., Kimball, A., Kini, U., Kline, A. D., Lauzon, J., Lildballe, D. L., López-González, V., Martinezmoles, J., Meldrum, C., Mirzaa, G. M., Morel, C. F., Morton, J. V., Pyle, L. C., Quintero-Rivera, F., Richer, J., Scheuerle, A. E., Bitten Schönewolf-Greulich, B., Shears, D. J., Josh Silver, J., Smith, A. C., I Karen Temple, K. I.; UCLA Clinical Genomics Center; van de Kamp, J. M., Fleur S van Dijk, F. S., Vandersteen, A. M., White, S. M., Zackai, E. H., Zou, R.; Care4Rare Canada Consortium; Bulman, D. E., Boycott, K. M., Matthew A Lines, M.A. 2016. "Mandibulofacial dysostosis with microcephaly: Mutation and database update." *Hum Mutat*, 37(2), 148-154. https://doi.org/10.1002/humu.22924.

Jones, Kenneth Lyons, Marilyn Crandall Jones and Miguel del Campo. 2013. *Smith's Recognizable Patterns of Human Malformation: Expert Consult - Online and Print*. 7th ed. Saunders.

Lines, M. A., Huang, L., Schwartzentruber, J., Douglas, S. L., Lynch, D. C., Beaulieu, C., Guion-Almeida, M. L., Roseli Maria Zechi-Ceide, R. M., Gener, B., Gillessen-Kaesbach, G., Nava, C., Baujat, G., Horn, D., Kini, U., Caliebe, A., Alanay, Y., Gulen Eda Utine, G. E., Lev, D., Kohlhase, J., Arthur W Grix, A. W., Lohmann, D. R., Hehr, U., Detlef

Böhm, D.; FORGE Canada Consortium; Majewski, J. Bulman, D. E., Dagmar Wieczorek, D., Boycott, K. M. 2012. "Haploinsufficiency of a spliceosomal GTPase encoded by EFTUD2 causes mandibulofacial dysostosis with microcephaly." *Am J Hum Genet*, 90(2), 369-377. https://doi.org/10.1016/j.ajhg.2011.12.023.

Luquetti, D. V., Hing, A. V., Rieder, M. J., Nickerson, D. A., Turner, E. H., Smith, J., Park, S., and Cunningham, M. L. 2013. "Mandibulofacial dysostosis with microcephaly caused by EFTUD2 mutations: expanding the phenotype." *Am J Med Genet A*, 161A(1), 108-113. Doi: https://doi.org/10.1002/ajmg.a.35696.

Online Mendelian Inheritance in Man (OMIM®). 2022. McKusick-Nathans Institute of Genetic Medicine, Johns Hopkins University (Baltimore, MD). World Wide Web URL: https://omim.org/

Wieczorek, D., Gener, B., González, MJ, Seland, S., Fischer, S., Hehr, U. Kuechler, A., Lies H Hoefsloot, L. H., Nicole de Leeuw, N., Gillessen-Kaesbach, G., Dietmar R Lohmann, D. R. 2009. "Microcephaly, microtia, preauricular tags, choanal atresia and developmental delay in three unrelated patients: a mandibulofacial dysostosis distinct from Treacher Collins Syndrome." *Am J Med Genet A*, 149A(5), 837-843. https://doi.org/10.1002/ajmg.a.32747.

Mandibulofacial dysostosis with alopecia

Mandibulofacial dysostosis with alopecia (OMIM 616367) is a rare condition observed in four individuals unrelated to *de novo* missense variants in the *EDNRA* gene. Clinically, the facial pattern of the individuals with mandibulofacial dysostosis with alopecia is characterized by lower eyelid coloboma, facial hypoplasia, cleft palate, micrognathia, ear anomaly and alopecia. The maxillary bone is atypically dysmorphic. Radiological findings were observed in three individuals with marked hypoplasia of the frontozygomatic region resulting in a very wide Tessier cleft number 8 (frontozygomatic cleft), which in the soft tissue resulted in marked macroblepharon. It also presented agenesis of the temporal portion of the zygomatic arch (zygomatic process of the temporal bone) and mandibular hypoplasia, and one individual was described by Cushman et al. (2005) as having depressions at the lateral aspects of the eyes, consistent with underlying lateral orbital anomalies (Zechi-Ceide et al. 2010; Gordon et al. 2015).

References

Cushman, L.J., Torres-Martinez, W., and Weaver, D.D. 2005. "Johnson-McMillin Syndrome: Report of a New Case with Novel Features." *Birth Defects Research Part A: Clinical and Molecular Teratology*, 73, 638-641. https://doi.org/10.1002/bdra.20178.

Gordon, CT., Weaver, KN., Zechi-Ceide, RM., Madsen, EC., Tavares, AL., Oufadem, M., Kurihara, Y., Adameyko, I., Picard, A., Breton, S., Pierrot, S., Biosse-Duplan, M., Voisin, N., Masson, C., Bole-Feysot, C., Nitschké, P., Delrue, MA., Lacombe, D., Guion-Almeida, ML., Moura, PP., Garib, DG., Munnich, A., Ernfors, P., Hufnagel, RB., Hopkin, RJ., Kurihara, H., Saal, HM., Weaver, DD., Katsanis, N., Lyonnet, S., Golzio, C., Clouthier, DE., Amiel, J. 2015. "Mutations in the endothelin receptor type A cause mandibulofacial dysostosis with alopecia." *American Journal of Human Genetics*, 96(4), 519-531. https://doi.org/10.1016/j.ajhg.2015.01.015.

Online Mendelian Inheritance in Man (OMIM®). 2022. McKusick-Nathans Institute of Genetic Medicine, Johns Hopkins University (Baltimore, MD). World Wide Web URL: https://omim.org/

Zechi-Ceide, R.M., Guion-Almeida, M.L., Jehee, F.S., Rocha, K., and Passos-Bueno, M.R. 2010. "Mandibulofacial dysostosis, severe lower eyelid coloboma, cleft palate, and alopecia: A new distinct form of mandibulofacial dysostosis or a severe form of Johnson-McMillin syndrome?" *American Journal of Medical Genetics Part A*, 152A, 1838-1840. https://doi.org/10.1002/ajmg.a.33477.

Acrofacial dysostosis

Nager syndrome

Nager syndrome (OMIM154400) is the most common form of acrofacial dysostosis. It was described by Nager and de Reynier in 1948. This rare condition has an autosomal dominant or recessive inheritance pattern, suggesting genetic heterogeneity. The Nager syndrome occurs due to the loss of function of pathogenic variants in the *SF3B4* gene, and some cases are likely due to a de novo variant (Nager and Reynier, 1948; Hennekam, Allanson and Krantz, 2010; Bernier et al. 2012; Terrazas et al. 2017; Beauchamp et al. 2020).

Clinically, it is characterized by down-slanting palpebral fissures, a flat nasal bridge, malar hypoplasia, maxillomandibular hypoplasia, a cleft palate, uvula atresia, limited mouth opening severe micrognathia, and abnormal ears (internal and external), overlapping the craniofacial phenotype of the Treacher Collins syndrome. The limb anomalies include hypoplasia or absence of the thumb, a short forearm, limitation of the elbow extension, proximal radioulnar synostosis and lower limb deformities. Other clinical features include short stature, respiratory distress, cardiac anomalies, costovertebral anomalies, intellectual disability, and microcephaly (Bozatlıoğlu and Münevveroğlu 2015; Rosa et al. 2015; Drozniewska et al. 2020).

Radiologically, it is characterized by mandibular and maxillary hypoplasia with Tessier cleft number 7 (temporozygomatic cleft), represented by a deficient zygomatic complex with a cleft in the zygomatic arch (Wu, Sakahara and Imai, 2017).

References

Beauchamp, M. C., Alam, S. S., Kumar, S., & Jerome-Majewska, L. A. 2020. "Spliceosomopathies and neurocristopathies: Two sides of the same coin?" *Developmental Dynamics*, 249(8), 924-945. https://doi.org/10.1002/dvdy.183.

Bernier FP, Caluseriu O, Ng S, Schwartzentruber J, Buckingham KJ, Innes AM, Jabs EW, Innis JW, Schuette JL, Gorski JL, Byers PH, Andelfinger G, Siu V, Lauzon J, Fernandez BA, McMillin M, Scott RH, Racher H; FORGE Canada Consortium; Majewski J, Nickerson DA, Shendure J, Bamshad MJ, Parboosingh JS. 2012. "Haploinsufficiency of SF3B4, a component of the pre-mRNA spliceosomal complex, causes Nager syndrome." *American Journal of Human Genetics* 90: 925.

https://doi.org/10.1016/j.ajhg.2012.04.004.
Bozatlıoğlu, R and Münevveroğlu, AP. 2015. "Dental Management of a Patient with Nager Acrofacial Dysostosis." *Case Reports in Dentistry* 2015: 984732. https://doi.org/10.1155/2015/984732.
Drozniewska M, Kilby MD, Vogt J, Togneri F, Quinlan-Jones E, Reali L, Allen S, McMullan D. 2020. "Second-trimester prenatal diagnosis of Nager syndrome with a deletion including SF3B4 detected by chromosomal microarray." *Clinical Case Reports* 8(3): 508-511. https://doi.org/10.1002/ccr3.2509.
Hennekam, Raoul, Judith E. Allanson, and Ian Krantz. 2010. *Gorlin's Syndromes of the Head and Neck*. 5th ed. New York, NY: Oxford University Press.
Jones, Kenneth Lyons, Marilyn Crandall Jones and Miguel del Campo. 2013. *Smith's Recognizable Patterns of Human Malformation: Expert Consult - Online and Print*. 7th ed. Saunders.
Nager, FR and de Reynier, JP. 1948. "Das Gehörorgan bei den angeborenen Kopfmissbildungen." *Pract Otorhinolaryngol* (Basal) 10 (Suppl 2): 1.
Online Mendelian Inheritance in Man (OMIM®). 2022. McKusick-Nathans Institute of Genetic Medicine, Johns Hopkins University (Baltimore, MD). World Wide Web URL: https://omim.org/
Rosa, R. F., Guimarães, V. B., Beltrão, L. A., Trombetta, J. S., Lliguin, K. L., de Mattos, V. F., & Zen, P. R. 2015. "Nager syndrome and Pierre Robin sequence." *Pediatric International*, 57(2), e69-e72. https://doi.org/10.1111/ped.12562.
Terrazas, K., Dixon, J., Trainor, P. A., & Dixon, M. J. 2017. "Rare syndromes of the head and face: mandibulofacial and acrofacial dysostoses." *Wiley Interdisciplinary Reviews: Developmental Biology*, 6(3), 10.1002/wdev.263. https://doi.org/10.1002/wdev.263.
Wu, CC, Sakahara, D and Imai, K. 2017. "Ankylosis of Temporomandibular Joints After Mandibular Distraction Osteogenesis in Patients with Nager Syndrome: Report of Two Cases and Literature Review." *Journal of Plastic, Reconstructive & Aesthetic Surgery* 70 (10): 1449-1456. https://doi.org/10.1016/j.bjps.2016.12.014

Richieri-Costa-Pereira Syndrome (RCPS)

The acrofacial dysostosis Richieri-Costa-Pereira syndrome (OMIM 268305) is an autosomal recessive condition, mainly described in Brazilian individuals, initially in 1992. Most of the families described were from a small geographical area in the southeast of Brazil, and the family history showed a high rate of recurrence in siblings/cousins, and the condition is causative by variants affecting the gene *EIF4A3* (Favaro et al. 2011; Lehalle et al. 2015; Bertola et al. 2018).

Classical phenotypes include microstomia, a cleft palate, Robin sequence, micrognathia, absent central lower incisors, median mandibular cleft (Tessier cleft number 30), minor ears anomalies, laryngeal anomalies, airway obstruction, feeding difficulties, and radial and tibial deficiencies associated with clubfeet (Favaro et al. 2014). Recent studies revealed a broad phenotypic spectrum within the RCPS reported in individuals with pathogenic variants in the *EIF4A3* gene, such as microcephaly, mild facial dysmorphisms, and an absent mandibular cleft (Bertola et al. 2018).

References

Bertola, D. R., Hsia, G., Alvizi, L., Gardham, A., Wakeling, E. L., Yamamoto, G. L., Honjo, R. S., Oliveira, L. A. N., Di Francesco, R. C., Perez, B. A., Kim, C. A., & Passos-Bueno, M. R. 2018. "Richieri-Costa-Pereira syndrome: Expanding its phenotypic and genotypic spectrum." *Clinical Genetics*, 93(4), 800-811. https://doi.org/10.1111/cge.13169.

Favaro, F. P., Alvizi, L., Zechi-Ceide, R. M., Bertola, D., Felix, T. M., de Souza, J., Raskin, S., Twigg, S. R., Weiner, A. M., Armas, P., Margarit, E., Calcaterra, N. B., Andersen, G. R., McGowan, S. J., Wilkie, A. O., Richieri-Costa, A., de Almeida, M. L., & Passos-Bueno, M. R. 2014. "A noncoding expansion in EIF4A3 causes Richieri-Costa-Pereira syndrome, a craniofacial disorder associated with limb defects." *American Journal of Human Genetics*, 94(1), 120-128. https://doi.org/10.1016/j.ajhg.2013.11.020.

Favaro, F. P., Zechi-Ceide, R. M., Alvarez, C. W., Maximino, L. P., Antunes, L. F., Richieri-Costa, A., & Guion-Almeida, M. L. 2011. "Richieri-Costa-Pereira syndrome: A unique acrofacial dysostosis type. An overview of the Brazilian cases." *American Journal of Medical Genetics Part A*, 155A(2), 322-331. https://doi.org/10.1002/ajmg.a.33806.

Online Mendelian Inheritance in Man (OMIM®). 2022. McKusick-Nathans Institute of Genetic Medicine, Johns Hopkins University (Baltimore, MD). World Wide Web URL: https://omim.org/

Lehalle, D., Wieczorek, D., Zechi-Ceide, R. M., Passos-Bueno, M. R., Lyonnet, S., Amiel, J., & Gordon, C. T. 2015. "A review of craniofacial disorders caused by spliceosomal defects." *Clinical Genetics*, 88(5), 405-415. https://doi.org/10.1111/cge.12596.

Syndrome of first and second pharyngeal arches

Oculoauriculovertebral Spectrum (OAVS)

Oculoauriculovertebral spectrum (OMIM 164210) is the most predominant condition represented by a deficiency in morphogenesis of the first and second pharyngeal arches affecting approximately 1:5600 individuals, and a prevalence of 3:2 is observed for males and the affected right side (Hennekam, Allanson and Krantz, 2010).

Cohen, Rollnick and Kaye (1989) described the term oculoauriculovertebral spectrum (OAVS) for the first time, and this complex condition is also known as hemifacial microsomia, Goldenhar syndrome or oculoauriculovertebral dysplasia (Cohen, Rollnick and Kaye 1989; Hennekam, Allanson and Krantz, 2010; Jones, Jones and Del Campo 2013).

Oculoauriculovertebral spectrum occurs sporadically in most cases, with a recurrence risk of 2%, except in cases where it is observed the presence of preauricular appendages and/or microtia in the family history, where the risk is increased (Hennekam, Allanson and Krantz, 2010; Beleza-Meireles et al. 2014; Evans, Hing and Cunningham, 2018)

Clinical phenotypes are highly variable and can affect one or both sides of the face (always asymmetric). The anomalies can affect feeding, compromise the airway, alter facial movement, disrupt hearing and alter facial appearance. The clinical features include coloboma of the upper eyelid, epibulbar dermoid, microphthalmia, hypoplasia of the mandible, malformation and ankylosis of the temporomandibular joint, paralysis of facial muscles, anomalies of the ears (external, middle and internal), and vertebral anomalies (such as scoliosis or hemivertebrae and cervical vertebrae). Less frequent features include cardiac and central nervous system anomalies (Hennekam, Allanson and Krantz, 2010; Beleza-Meireles et al., 2014; Birgfeld and Heike, 2019).

The phenotype of OAVS and its severity may depend on the expression and activation of genes during facial development, and variable expressivity makes its molecular diagnosis difficult. Therefore, the asymmetrical facial phenotype of OAVS and other syndromes involving facial bone alterations may become more evident with craniofacial growth. (Beleza-Meireles et al. 2014; Tingaud-Sequeira et al. 2022).

Molecular studies identified genes that are related to the oculoauriculovertebral spectrum. One study evaluated 169 individuals with clinical findings compatible with this condition and found variants in the *MYT1* gene (Lopez et al. 2016; Zamariolli et al. 2021). Recently, another study showed that haploinsufficiency of the *SF3B2* gene is responsible for the cause of OAVS, both in sporadic and familial recurrence cases (Timberlake et al. 2021).

Bone anomalies are frequently described, including rare facial clefts. The most common rare cleft in OAVS is the Tessier cleft number 7 in soft tissue (lateral oral cleft that results in macrostomia). This cleft also affects the bone, characterized by a temporozygomatic cleft (in a zygomatic arch) that can occur along with other anomalies, such as maxillary duplication and posterior maxillary clefts (Chauhan, Guruprasad 2015; Timberlake et al. 2021). Other less frequent clefts were reported in cases with the oculoauriculovertebral spectrum, such as the paramedian mandibular cleft, also known as the Tessier cleft number 30 (Tanna et al. 2012; Vendramini-Pittoli et al. 2015).

References

Beleza-Meireles, Ana, Jill Clayton-Smith, Jorge M. Saraiva, and May Tassabehji. 2014. "Oculo-Auriculo-Vertebral Spectrum: A Review of the Literature and Genetic Update." *Journal of Medical Genetics* 51 (10): 635–45. https://doi.org/10.1136/jmedgenet-2014-102476.

Birgfeld, Craig and Carrie Heike. 2019. "Craniofacial Microsomia." *Clinics in Plastic Surgery* 46 (2): 207–21. https://doi.org/10.1016/j.cps.2018.12.001.

Chauhan, Dinesh Singh and Yadavalli Guruprasad. 2015. "Bilateral Tessier's 7 Cleft with Maxillary Duplication." *Journal of Maxillofacial and Oral Surgery* 14 (S1): 108–12. https://doi.org/10.1007/s12663-012-0346-x.

Cohen, M. M., B. R. Rollnick, and C. I. Kaye. 1989. "Oculoauriculovertebral Spectrum: An Updated Critique." *Cleft Palate J* 26 (4): 276–86.

Evans, Kelly N., Anne V. Hing, and Michael L. Cunningham. 2018. "Craniofacial Malformations." In *Avery's Diseases of the Newborn*, 1417-1437.e2. Elsevier.

Hennekam, Raoul, Judith E. Allanson, and Ian Krantz. 2010. *Gorlin's Syndromes of the Head and Neck*. 5th ed. New York, NY: Oxford University Press.

Jones, Kenneth Lyons, Marilyn Crandall Jones and Miguel del Campo. 2013. *Smith's Recognizable Patterns of Human Malformation: Expert Consult - Online and Print*. 7th ed. Saunders.

Lopez, Estelle, Marie Berenguer, Angèle Tingaud-Sequeira, Sandrine Marlin, Annick Toutain, Françoise Denoyelle, Arnaud Picard, et al. 2016. "Mutations inMYT1, Encoding the Myelin Transcription Factor 1, Are a Rare Cause of OAVS." *Journal of Medical Genetics* 53 (11): 752–60. https://doi.org/10.1136/jmedgenet-2016-103774.

Online Mendelian Inheritance in Man (OMIM®). 2022. McKusick-Nathans Institute of Genetic Medicine, Johns Hopkins University (Baltimore, MD). World Wide Web URL: https://omim.org/

Tanna, Neil, Derrick C. Wan, Adam D. Perry, Henry K. Kawamoto, and James P. Bradley. 2012. "Paramedian Mandibular Cleft: Revisiting the Tessier Classification." *The Journal of Craniofacial Surgery* 23 (1): e38–40. https://doi.org/10.1097/scs.0b013e318241db58.

Timberlake, Andrew T., Casey Griffin, Carrie L. Heike, Anne V. Hing, Michael L. Cunningham, David Chitayat, Mark R. Davis, et al. 2021. "Haploinsufficiency of SF3B2 Causes Craniofacial Microsomia." *Nature Communications* 12 (1). https://doi.org/10.1038/s41467-021-24852-9.

Tingaud-Sequeira, Angèle, Aurélien Trimouille, Thomas Sagardoy, Didier Lacombe and Caroline Rooryck. 2022. "Oculo-Auriculo-Vertebral Spectrum: New Genes and Literature Review on a Complex Disease." *Journal of Medical Genetics* 59 (5): 417–27. https://doi.org/10.1136/jmedgenet-2021-108219.

Vendramini-Pittoli, Siulan, Maria L. Guion-Almeida, Juliana M. Santos, Silvio M. Garcia Júnior, Mauricio M. Yoshida, Antonio Richieri-Costa and Nancy M. Kokitsu-Nakata. 2015. "An Unusual Presentation of Oculoauriculovertebral Spectrum with a Tessier 30 Cleft: Report on Two Cases." *Clinical Dysmorphology* 24 (4): 144–50. https://doi.org/10.1097/mcd.0000000000000085.

Zamariolli, Malú, Bruna Burssed, Mariana Moysés-Oliveira, Mileny Colovati, Fernanda Teixeira da Silva Bellucco, Leonardo Caires Santos, Ana Beatriz Alvarez Perez, Silvia Bragagnolo and Maria Isabel Melaragno. 2021. "Novel MYT1 Variants Expose the Complexity of Oculo-auriculo-vertebral Spectrum Genetic Mechanisms." *American Journal of Medical Genetics*. Part A 185 (7): 2056–64. https://doi.org/10.1002/ajmg.a.62217.

Complex conditions with Tessier Clefts

Amniotic band sequence

Amniotic band sequence is also called congenital constriction bands, amniotic bands, or amniotic band syndrome (OMIM 217100). Many different classifications have been proposed in the literature. It has been considered a multifactorial condition that may involve three basic types of anomalies, including malformations, deformations and disruptions resulting in a complex group congenital anomaly. Some disruptive factors and malformations cannot be explained embryologically (Torpin, 1968; Hennekam, Allanson and Krantz, 2010; Doğru and Ali Acar, 2023).

The amnion rupture and small strands of amnion can encircle developing structures resulting in ring constrictions intrauterine and multiple congenital anomalies that affect the head and neck, such as an asymmetric central nervous system, craniofacial clefts, body wall deficiency (including gastrointestinal and cardiovascular system), limb reduction, and amputations in many cases (Coady, Moore and Wallis, 1998; Jones, Marko and Del Campo 2013; López-Muñoz and Becerra-Solano, 2018). However, the origin of the amniotic band is unclear, and the clinical signs are variable; in some severe conditions, the central nervous system and cardiovascular anomalies are involved, and perinatal mortality may occur (Waterson, 1982; Sadler, 2014).

Recurrence of this condition is rare, and genetic analysis is not typically recommended because the cases generally are sporadic (Gandhi, Rac, McKinney 2019). Different risk factors have been reported in the literature, but no risk factor was consistently found (Bergman et al. 2022; Doğru and Ali Acar 2023).

Lowry, Bedard and Sibbald, 2016 performed a study of the prevalence of clinical findings related to amniotic band sequence and described some associations with anencephaly, encephalocele, Tessier clefts, cleft lip with or without cleft palate, and cleft palate only. In another group, amniotic band sequences were observed with some limb deficiencies that include the absence or hypoplasia of a limb or part of a limb, digital deficiencies and craniofacial anomalies, such as one group with anencephaly, encephalocele, anophthalmia, nose malformations, Tessier clefts, cleft lip with or without cleft palate. Another group reported amniotic band sequences with ring constrictions, craniofacial anomalies, failure to form the body wall and limb malformations with absence or hypoplasia (Lies et al. 2019).

In most cases of amniotic band sequence, the multiple Tessier clefts are usually asymmetric. Complex cases cannot be explained because they do not observe a classical pattern of anomalies (López-Muñoz and Becerra-Solano, 2018).

In a retrospective review, Lies et al. (2019) reported that major craniofacial anomalies cannot be completely explained based on the premature amniotic layer, which suggests a multifactoral condition.

References

Bergman, Jorieke E. H., Ingeborg Barišić, Marie-Claude Addor, Paula Braz, Clara Cavero-Carbonell, Elizabeth S. Draper, Luis J. Echevarría-González-de-Garibay, et al. 2022. "Amniotic Band Syndrome and Limb Body Wall Complex in Europe 1980–2019." *American Journal of Medical Genetics. Part A*. https://doi.org/10.1002/ajmg.a.63107.

Coady, M. S., M. H. Moore, and K. Wallis. 1998. "Amniotic Band Syndrome: The Association between Rare Facial Clefts and Limb Ring Constrictions." *Plast Reconstr Surg* 101 (3): 640–49. https://doi.org/10.1097/00006534-199803000-00010.

Cohen, M. Michael. 2006. *Perspectives on the Face*. New York, NY: Oxford University Press.

Doğru, Şükran and Ali Acar. 2023. "Fetoscopic Surgery for Amniotic Band Syndrome: Case Series." *Congenital Anomalies* 63 (1): 4–8. https://doi.org/10.1111/cga.12494.

Gandhi, Manisha, Martha W. F. Rac, and Jennifer McKinney. 2019. "Amniotic Band Sequence." *American Journal of Obstetrics and Gynecology* 221 (6): B5–6. https://doi.org/10.1016/j.ajog.2019.09.020.

Hennekam, Raoul, Judith E. Allanson, and Ian Krantz. 2010. *Gorlin's Syndromes of the Head and Neck*. 5th ed. New York, NY: Oxford University Press.

Jones, Kenneth Lyons, Marilyn Crandall Jones and Miguel del Campo. 2013. *Smith's Recognizable Patterns of Human Malformation*: Expert Consult - Online and Print. 7th ed. Saunders.

Lies, Shelby, Terri Beckwith, Janith Mills, Lesley Butler, Marybeth Ezaki and Scott Oishi. 2019. "Case Series: Amniotic Band Sequence with Craniofacial Abnormalities." *Birth Defects Research* 111 (19): 1494–1500. https://doi.org/10.1002/bdr2.1576.

López-Muñoz, E., and L. E. Becerra-Solano. 2018. "An Update on Amniotic Bands Sequence." *Arch Argent Pediatr* 116 (3): e409–20. https://doi.org/ 10.5546/aap.2018.eng.e409.

Lowry, R. B., T. Bedard, and B. Sibbald. 2016. "The Prevalence of Amnion Rupture Sequence, Limb Body Wall Defects and Body Wall Defects in Alberta 1980-2012 with a Review of Risk Factors and Familial Cases." *Am J Med Genet Part A* 9999: 1–10. https://doi.org/ 10.1002/ajmg.a.38016.

Online Mendelian Inheritance in Man (OMIM®). 2022. McKusick-Nathans Institute of Genetic Medicine, Johns Hopkins University (Baltimore, MD). World Wide Web URL: https://omim.org/.

Sadler, T. W. 2014. *Langman's Medical Embryology*. 13th ed. Philadelphia, PA: Lippincott Williams and Wilkins.

Torpin, R. 1968. *Fetal malformations caused by amnion rupture during gestation*. Thomas. Springfield, Ill.: Charles C Thomas (pub.) 1968.

Waterson, J. R. 1982. *The Child with Multiple Birth Defects M. Michael Cohen*. New York: Jr. Raven Press.

CHAPTER NINETEEN

THE APPLICATION OF COMPUTED TOMOGRAPHY IN CRANIOFACIAL CLINICAL PRACTICE

Medical imaging techniques are currently used in large craniofacial treatment and research centres, including magnetic resonance imaging and computed tomography, to estimate craniofacial malformations. This is of great importance in the prenatal diagnosis of these conditions and for evaluating pre and postoperative malformations. (Garel et al., 2021; Gosla Reddy and Acharya, 2021).

The diagnosis by image has been used to aid clinical diagnosis, enabling a more accurate morphological assessment of the craniofacial region (Mehrotra et al. 2011). Three-dimensional (3D) image analysis provides higher quality and more detailed information than conventional two-dimensional (2D) radiography, aiding the differential diagnosis. Reference Craniofacial Centres have been using resources such as 2D and 3D imaging, including computed tomography scan (CT), magnetic resonance imaging (MRI) and 3D photogrammetry for planning and executing treatment of the craniofacial complex associated with clinical-genetic evaluation (Cox, Luquetti and Cunningham 2013; Anderson et al. 2014; Pellerin 2022).

In the last two decades, with the increased use of three-dimensional (3D) images to evaluate maxillofacial morphology, cone beam computed tomography has also been chosen for this assessment because it provides a lower radiation dose than the helical CT, and it allows evaluation of the midface, jaw and/or temporomandibular joint, facial asymmetry, and craniofacial growth regions (Caruso, Harris and Padwa, 2003; Kapila, Conley and Harrell, 2011; Cox, Luquetti and Cunningham 2013; Anderson et al. 2014; Garib et al. 2014 Kaasalainen et al. 2021).

Cone beam tomography (CBCT) allows the visualization of craniofacial morphology in multiplanar sections (axial, coronal and sagittal) with high resolution. It presents clinical evidence for craniofacial evaluation and for planning the treatment of orofacial clefts, craniofacial clefts, craniofacial syndromes, skeletal discrepancies, temporomandibular joint pathologies and analysing the craniofacial complex at different angles since planning using this technology improves the therapeutic approach for maxillofacial deformities (Garib et al. 2007; Anderson et al. 2014; Garib et al. 2014; Kapila and Nervina, 2015).

Radiological Evaluation in Craniofacial Syndromes

The first reports on the use of 3D computed tomography in patients with craniofacial anomalies were realized in 1989 by Marsh and Vannier. The authors showed that the use of this technology helped in the study of craniofacial anomalies and that the 3D image reconstructions have already helped in the differentiation of similar phenotypes. David, Moore, and Cooter 1989 evaluated the craniofacial morphology of Tessier's clefts using third-dimensional computed tomography (CT) reconstruction, which showed more accurate details, to delineate clefts in bone tissue.

Subsequently, Posnick, Goldstein and Waitzman (1993) evaluated deficiencies in the zygomatic complex in children with Treacher Collins syndrome. Darling et al. (1994) proved the efficacy of 3D CT over 2D CT, evaluating patients with craniosynostosis, rare facial clefts, trauma and craniofacial syndromes.

Johnson et al. (2011) evaluated some first and second pharyngeal arch syndromes, including individuals with Robin sequence, hemifacial microsomia and auriculocondylar syndrome. In patients with Robin sequence, radiographic evaluation showed symmetrical mandibular hypoplasia, which may be associated with hypoplasia of the condylar process and coronoid process.

Radiological evaluation with 3D reconstruction in individuals with hemifacial microsomia showed variable involvement of facial structures (which may affect only one side of the face), such as hypoplasia and asymmetry of the maxilla and mandible and malformation of the temporomandibular joint. The authors also reported that detailed examinations of the temporal bone should be considered to assess the middle ear and the formation of the facial nerve, to classify the severity of each craniofacial manifestation of microsomia hemifacial (Johnson et al. 2011).

The 3D CT reconstruction of individuals with Goldenhar syndrome allows the volumetric reproduction of anatomical structures of the skull without superimposition, enabling a complete evaluation of all the malformations present in the mandible and temporal bone, which characterize the syndrome and help in the conduction of the therapy and orthodontic treatment (Saccomanno et al. 2014).

In Stickler's syndrome, a low nasal bridge, mild hypoplasia of the zygomatic bone, micrognathia, temporal bone evaluation and anomalies in the ossicular chain were also observed in radiographic evaluation. Morphological findings show that understanding these anomalies' radiological findings helps formulate accurate diagnoses and consider differential diagnoses (Johnson et al. 2011).

Among the morphologically evaluated mandibulofacial dysostosis, Treacher Collins syndrome, which has been evaluated by cephalometric analysis and computed tomography, aiming a better characterization of anomalies and improvement in surgical results overlapping facial features and dysfunctions associated with this condition (Chong et al. 2008; Chung et al. 2012; Kapadia et al. 2013; Wong et al. 2013). 3D morphological analysis was also performed to compare the mandible of individuals with Treacher Collins syndrome and individuals with Robin Sequence (Chung et al. 2012; Kato et al. 2021).

Wong et al. (2013), using 3D CT, identified different degrees of malar hypoplasia in individuals with Treacher Collins syndrome and classified the findings as mild, moderate and severe. The authors also observed that the right and left sides are not symmetrically affected.

Luquetti et al. (2013) performed a molecular and radiological study on three individuals with Guion-Almeida-type MFD. They observed that evaluating a cleft in the zygomatic arch in 3D CT helps in the differential diagnosis of clinical signs overlapping the oculoauriculovertebral spectrum with bilateral microtia. They found pathogenic variants in *EFTUD2* in all individuals and added a cleft zygomatic arch and epibulbar dermoid to the clinical phenotype. The authors suggest that studies of craniofacial images of the zygomatic arch could help diagnose Guion-Almeida-type MFD.

In another study with MFD Guion-Almeida type, Sarkar et al. (2015) evaluated two individuals with middle and inner ear alterations through a temporal bone CT; their findings expanded the phenotype and helped in the differential diagnosis since these findings overlap the findings observed in CHARGE syndrome.

Moura et al. (2017) performed a phenotypic refinement in a clinical and radiological study on a sample of mandibulofacial dysostosis, a rare condition described by Marçano and Richieri-Costa (1998) in a Brazilian family. Until now, eleven cases have been described; recurrence was observed in two out of eight families, and the affected distribution pattern was compatible with autosomal dominant inheritance in one and autosomal recessive in the other, indicating possible genetic heterogeneity for this condition. The clinical phenotype was characterized by severe underdevelopment of the mandible, midface hypoplasia, orofacial cleft, bitemporal narrowing, a mildly down-slanting upper eyelid, a high nasal bridge, thick and everted lower lip, minor ears abnormalities and hearing loss. Radiographic aspects included down slanting of the zygomatic arch, maxillary hypoplasia, microretrognathia, hypoplastic mandibular condyles and an ectopic external auditory canal. The inclination of the zygomatic arch, present in 100% of the individuals studied, has not been reported in other conditions with MFD, seeming to be a specific finding of mandibulofacial dysostosis Bauru type. Due to the rarity of human facial dysostosis, the three-dimensional radiographic studies are small. However, the reported data show the importance of characterizing the facial alterations in this condition to understand the facial malformation's presence better, allowing a more accurate diagnosis and personalized treatment plan.

References

Anderson, P. J., R. Yong, T. L. Surman, Z. A. Rajion, and S. Ranjitkar. 2014. "Application of Three-Dimensional Computed Tomography in Craniofacial Clinical Practice and Research". *Australian Dental Journal* 59 Suppl 1: 174–85. https://doi.org/10.1111/adj.12154.

Caruso, Paul A., Gordon J. Harris, and Bonnie L. Padwa. 2003. "CT Imaging of Craniofacial Malformations". *Neuroimaging Clinics of North America* 13 (3): 541–72. https://doi.org/10.1016/s1052-5149(03)00061-3.

Chong, David K., Dylan J. Murray, Jonathan A. Britto, Brian Tompson, Christopher R. Forrest, and John H. Phillips. 2008. "A Cephalometric Analysis of Maxillary and Mandibular Parameters in Treacher Collins Syndrome". *Plastic and Reconstructive Surgery* 121 (3): 77e–84e. https://doi.org/10.1097/01.prs.0000299379.64906.2e.

Chung, Michael T., Benjamin Levi, Jeong S. Hyun, David D. Lo, Daniel T. Montoro, Jeffrey Lisiecki, James P. Bradley, Steven R. Buchman, Michael T. Longaker, and Derrick C. Wan. 2012. "Pierre Robin Sequence and Treacher Collins Hypoplastic Mandible Comparison

Using Three-Dimensional Morphometric Analysis". *The Journal of Craniofacial Surgery* 23 (7 Suppl 1): 1959–63. https://doi.org/10.1097/SCS.0b013e318258bcf1.

Cox, Timothy C., Daniela V. Luquetti, and Michael L. Cunningham. 2013. "Perspectives and Challenges in Advancing Research into Craniofacial Anomalies: AMERICAN JOURNAL OF MEDICAL GENETICS PART C (SEMINARS IN MEDICAL GENETICS)". *American Journal of Medical Genetics. Part C, Seminars in Medical Genetics* 163C (4): 213–17. https://doi.org/10.1002/ajmg.c.31383.

Darling, C. F., S. E. Byrd, E. D. Allen, M. A. Radkowski, and M. A. Wilczynski. 1994. "Three-Dimensional Computed Tomography Imaging in the Evaluation of Craniofacial Abnormalities". *Journal of the National Medical Association* 86 (9): 676–80.

Garel, Catherine, Saskia Vande Perre, Lucie Guilbaud, Véronique Soupre, Eléonore Blondiaux and Hubert Ducou le Pointe. 2021. "Contribution of Computed Tomography and Magnetic Resonance Imaging in the Analysis of Fetal Craniofacial Malformations". *Pediatric Radiology* 51 (10): 1917–28. https://doi.org/10.1007/s00247-021-05033-8.

Garib, Daniela G., Louise Resti Calil, Claudia Resende Leal, and Guilherme Janson. 2014. "Is There a Consensus for CBCT Use in Orthodontics?" *Dental Press Journal of Orthodontics* 19 (5): 136–49. https://doi.org/10.1590/2176-9451.19.5.136-149.sar.

Gosla Reddy, Srinivas, and Avni Pandey Acharya. 2021. "Rare Facial Clefts". Em *Oral and Maxillofacial Surgery for the Clinician*, 1735–68. Singapore: Springer Nature Singapore.

Johnson, J. M., G. Moonis, G. E. Green, R. Carmody, and H. N. Burbank. 2011. "Syndromes of the first and second branchial arches, part 1: embryology and characteristics defects". *AJNR Am J Neuroradiol* 32 (1): 14–19.

Kaasalainen, Touko, Marja Ekholm, Teemu Siiskonen and Mika Kortesniemi. 2021. "Dental Cone Beam CT: An Updated Review". *Physica Medica: PM: An International Journal Devoted to the Applications of Physics to Medicine and Biology: Official Journal of the Italian Association of Biomedical Physics (AIFB)* 88: 193–217. https://doi.org/10.1016/j.ejmp.2021.07.007.

Kadakia, Sameep, Samuel N. Helman, Arvind K. Badhey, Masoud Saman, and Yadranko Ducic. 2014. "Treacher Collins Syndrome: The Genetics of a Craniofacial Disease". *International Journal of Pediatric Otorhinolaryngology* 78 (6): 893–98. https://doi.org/10.1016/j.ijporl.2014.03.006.

Kapila, S., R. S. Conley, and W. E. Harrell Jr. 2011. "The Current Status of Cone Beam Computed Tomography Imaging in Orthodontics". *Dento Maxillo Facial Radiology* 40 (1): 24–34. https://doi.org/10.1259/dmfr/12615645.

Kapila, S. D., and J. M. Nervina. 2015. "CBCT in Orthodontics: Assessment of Treatment Outcomes and Indications for Its Use". *Dento Maxillo Facial Radiology* 44 (1): 20140282. https://doi.org/10.1259/dmfr.20140282.

Kato, Renata Mayumi, Priscila Padilha Moura, Roseli Maria Zechi-Ceide, Cristiano Tonello, Adriano Porto Peixoto and Daniela Garib. 2021. "Comparison between Treacher Collins Syndrome and Pierre Robin Sequence: A Cephalometric Study". *The Cleft Palate-Craniofacial Journal: Official Publication of the American Cleft Palate-Craniofacial Association* 58 (1): 78–83. https://doi.org/10.1177/1055665620937499.

Luquetti, D. V., A. V. Hing, M. J. Rieder, D. A. Nickerson, E. H. Turner, and J. Smith. 2013. "Mandibulofacial dysostosis with microcephaly" caused by EFTUD2 mutations: expanding the phenotype". *Am J Med Genet A* 161 (1): 108–13.

Marsh, J. L., and M. W. Vannier. 1989. "Three-Dimensional Surface Imaging from CT Scans for the Study of Craniofacial Dysmorphology". *Journal of Craniofacial Genetics and Developmental Biology* 9 (1): 61–75.

Mehrotra, Divya, Mahdi Hasan, Rahul Pandey, and Sumit Kumar. 2011. "Clinical Spectrum of Treacher Collins Syndrome." Journal of Oral Biology and Craniofacial Research 1 (1): 36–40. https://doi.org/10.1016/s2212-4268(11)60009-2.

Moura, Priscila P., Nancy M. Kokitsu-Nakata, Marília S. Yatabe, Siulan Vendramini-Pittoli, Pedro H. Hori, Maria L. Guion-Almeida, Daniela G. Garib, Antonio Richieri-Costa, and Roseli M. Zechi-Ceide. 2017. "Mandibulofacial Dysostosis Bauru Type: Refining the Phenotype". *American Journal of Medical Genetics. Part A* 173 (7): 1747–53. https://doi.org/10.1002/ajmg.a.38257.

Nardi, Cosimo, Luisa De Falco, Valeria Selvi, Chiara Lorini, Linda Calistri and Stefano Colagrande. 2018. "Role of Cone-Beam Computed Tomography with a Large Field of View in Goldenhar Syndrome". *American Journal of Orthodontics and Dentofacial Orthopedics: Official Publication of the American Association of Orthodontists, Its Constituent Societies, and the American Board of Orthodontics* 153 (2): 269–77. https://doi.org/10.1016/j.ajodo.2017.06.024.

Pellerin, Philippe. 2022. "Management of Hypertelorism". *Journal of Pediatric Neurosciences* 17 (5): 4. https://doi.org/10.4103/jpn.jpn_43_22.

Posnick, J. C., J. A. Goldstein, and A. A. Waitzman. 1993. "Surgical Correction of the Treacher Collins Malar Deficiency: Quantitative CT Scan Analysis of Long-Term Results". *Plastic and Reconstructive Surgery* 92 (1): 12–22. https://doi.org/10.1097/00006534-199307000-00002.

Saccomanno, S., F. Greco, L. D'Alatri, E. De Corso, M. Pandolfini, B. Sergi, T. Pirronti, and R. Deli. 2014. "Role of 3D-CT for Orthodontic and ENT Evaluation in Goldenhar Syndrome". *Acta Otorhinolaryngologica Italica: Organo Ufficiale Della Societa Italiana Di Otorinolaringologia e Chirurgia Cervico-Facciale* 34 (4): 283–87.

Sarkar, Arindam, Lisa T. Emrick, Eboni M. Smith, Elise G. Austin, Yaping Yang, Jill V. Hunter, Fernando Scaglia, and Seema R. Lalani. 2015. "Novel de Novo Mutations in EFTUD2 Detected by Exome Sequencing in Mandibulofacial Dysostosis with Microcephaly Syndrome: Novel de Novo mutations In EFTUD2". *American Journal of Medical Genetics. Part A* 167A (4): 914–18. https://doi.org/10.1002/ajmg.a.36948.